Farr's
Physics for
Medical Imaging

Farr's Physics for Medical Imaging

Third Edition

Alim Yucel-Finn MBBS, MSc, FRCR
Consultant Radiologist,
University Hospitals of North Midlands, UK

Fergus McKiddie PhD, MPE, MIPEM
Consultant Medical Physicist, Nuclear Medicine,
Aberdeen Royal Infirmary, Aberdeen, UK

Sarah Prescott MSci, MSc, MIPEM, MRSE (MRSC™)
Lead MRI Clinical Scientist and MR Safety Expert (MRSC™),
University Hospitals of North Midlands, UK

Rachel Griffiths MA, MSc
MRI and Ultrasound Clinical Scientist,
University Hospitals of North Midlands, UK

ELSEVIER

Notices

Practitioners and researchers must always rely on their own experience and knowledge in evaluating and using any information, methods, compounds or experiments described herein. Because of rapid advances in the medical sciences, in particular, independent verification of diagnoses and drug dosages should be made. To the fullest extent of the law, no responsibility is assumed by Elsevier, authors, editors or contributors for any injury and/or damage to persons or property as a matter of products liability, negligence or otherwise, or from any use or operation of any methods, products, instructions, or ideas contained in the material herein.

ISBN: 978-0-7020-8364-8

Content Strategist: Alexandra Mortimer
Content Project Manager: Fariha Nadeem
Illustration Manager: Nijantha Priyadharshini
Marketing Manager: Deborah Watkins

Printed in India

Last digit is the print number: 9 8 7 6 5 4 3 2 1

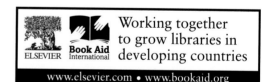

This title was first published in 1996, with the second edition coming out in 2008. The world of medical imaging, and thus radiology, has manifestly changed since then. Whilst analogue systems and the presence of radiology film were the standard in 1996, there are now consultant radiologists who have never encountered film in their working life. This book is aimed at those undertaking the FRCR part 1 physics examination, as it has always been, and the content has been updated to reflect the latest syllabus available. The biggest content change from the previous edition is the removal of analogue imaging techniques. These may still be in use worldwide, but for those in training in the United Kingdom, these are considered obsolete.

Whilst medical imaging has changed and evolved since the first edition, there are two other major sources of change during that time. The first is the take-off of artificial intelligence and computer-assisted radiology. There has been exponential growth in this industry, with untold products and services now marketed and developed. Whilst the underlying physics will not change, the interpretation of images, including their presentation and manipulation by algorithms before a human observes these images, will no doubt change. The second source of change has been COVID-19, a virus that has affected everyone. Compared to other medical colleagues, diagnostic radiologists have been comparatively luckier with the ability for remote reporting and teleconferencing facilitated by our digital infrastructure.

A great effort was made during the construction of this book to ease readability for understanding and recall, including the addition of more pictures. The underlying material however does not always facilitate this. A new chapter on radiology information technology was introduced to convey a number of concepts that are central to digital radiology. Too few radiologists can be considered IT 'super-users', and it is hoped that the introduction of the concepts in this chapter will inspire readers to further their own understanding and use of technology central to their working lives.

The authors would like to thank Mr. Sam Butler and Dr Abdel Kader Allouni for their help with proofreading and content review. The authors would also like to thank Dr Qamar Sharif and Dr Hussein Hassan for their reviews. The authors would also like to thank Siemens Healthcare Ltd. for allowing the use of pictures of their equipment. We also thank Alexandra Mortimer, Fariha Nadeem, and the staff at Elsevier for helping us through this book, particularly in the challenging times of COVID-19.

Matter and Radiation

CHAPTER CONTENTS

Diagnostic imaging is facilitated with the use of ionising and non-ionising radiations. Ionising radiations involve X- and gamma rays. Non-ionising radiations involve radio-frequency and sound. The body is partly transparent to these radiations, but not completely, and the interactions of these radiations with the body elements and compounds yield diagnostic imaging.

ATOMIC STRUCTURE

Matter is composed of atoms. Each atom is defined by its central nucleus. This contributes the majority of the mass. The nucleus is composed of nucleons: protons and neutrons. Protons have a relative mass of 1, with a +1 charge. Neutrons have a relative mass of 1, with 0 charge. Each nucleus is held together by a strong nuclear force.

The nucleons combine to yield the mass number of the atom. The number of protons determines the atomic number. This further defines the position of an atom in the periodic table and is synonymous with the name of the element. The number of associated neutrons can vary, yielding isotopes. These atoms have the same atomic number (number of protons) but a different number of neutrons. Some of these isotopes are unstable and decay with the emission of ionising radiation or particles (or both), called radioisotopes (see section on Radioactivity further on).

^{1}H is hydrogen. This contains only a proton with no neutron (see Fig. 1.1). ^{2}H (deuterium) and ^{3}H (tritium) are isotopes of hydrogen with neutrons.

^{12}C, ^{13}C, and ^{14}C are all carbon atoms with six protons (see Fig. 1.2). The ^{12}C diagram shows 6 orbiting electrons but in a specific arrangement. This arrangement is defined by the electron shells.

The nucleus is surrounded by shells of orbiting electrons. Each electron has a relative mass of 0.0005, with a −1 charge. The number of electrons usually matches the number of protons to balance the charge in the atom. There is a specific arrangement to electron shells. The innermost shell is termed the K-shell and can hold two electrons. Next is the L-shell, which holds eight electrons. The next shell, M, can hold 18 electrons, with the N shell holding 32 electrons. An example of sodium/Na is shown in Fig. 1.3.

Each of these shells has a varying number of subshells contributing to the overall shell, which also can influence the behaviour of electrons, but that is beyond the scope of this book [Further reading: Aufbau principle].

The outermost electron shell is referred to as the valence shell. The valence shell defines the chemical, thermal, optical, and electrical properties of the element. The valence shell can only ever have eight electrons within it (complete outer shell octet based on subshells).

Metals often have 1−3 valence electrons which can be easily detached from the atom, yielding nucleons within a 'sea of electrons.' They are good conductors of heat and electricity (see Fig. 1.4).

Valence shell electrons can also be shared between elements through a covalent bond yielding a crystal lattice (see Fig. 1.5). The lattice is held together by electrostatic attraction.

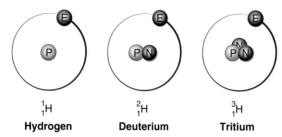

$${}^{1}_{1}\text{H}$$
Hydrogen

$${}^{2}_{1}\text{H}$$
Deuterium

$${}^{3}_{1}\text{H}$$
Tritium

Fig. 1.1 Nuclei and electron shells of the atoms of (A) hydrogen, (B) deuterium, and (C) tritium. (Original image: Image ID 1555863596 from www.Shutterstock.com)

Electrons are bound to shells based on binding energy. This binding energy is required to remove the electron from the attractive force of the nucleus (expressed in electronvolts, eV). Each shell has different binding energies, with $E_K > E_L > E_M$, etc. Each binding energy is fixed for a given element and shell level. When an inner shell electron is excited through the external deposition of energy, it can be raised to a higher electron shell. When the electron returns to its original shell, the excess energy is re-emitted as a photon. The energy value of the photon is consistent for each element, yielding characteristic photons (termed X-rays).

See Tables 1.1 and 1.2.

ELECTROMAGNETIC RADIATION

This is the umbrella term for energy travelling across empty space. All forms of electromagnetic (EM) radiation travel at the same velocity as light when in vacuo (2.98×10^8 ms^{-1}, similar in air).

EM radiation is considered to have both wave and particle-like properties, determined from the double slit experiment.

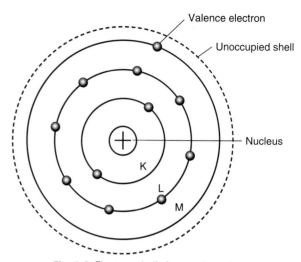

Fig. 1.3 Electron shells in a sodium atom.

From the quantum aspect, EM radiation can be considered as particles, represented as photons (quantised packets of energy).

From the wave aspect, EM radiation can also be considered as sinusoidally varying electric and magnetic fields. The electric and magnetic vectors are perpendicular to each other and perpendicular to the direction of the wave. Fig. 1.6 shows a wave of field strength vs time (can be considered a sine wave), where A = amplitude and T = time interval between successive wave crests. This yields:

$$\text{Frequency} = 1/T$$
$$\lambda f = c$$

where λ = wavelength, f = frequency, and c = constant (usually velocity). The EM spectrum is divided based on wavelength and frequency (see Table 1.3).

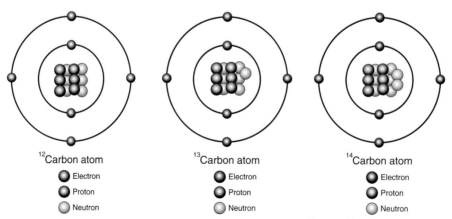

Fig. 1.2 Nuclei and electron shells of the carbon atoms: (A) ^{12}C, (B) ^{13}C, and (C) ^{14}C.

Metallic bonding

Electrons move freely along the sample

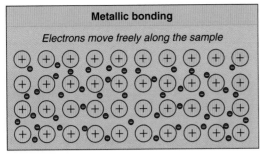

Fig. 1.4 Sea of electrons around metal atoms.

Silver (I) bromide

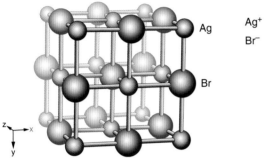

Ag
Br

Ag$^+$
Br$^-$

Fig. 1.5 Crystal lattice structure for silver bromide.

TABLE 1.2 Atomic Number (Z) and K-shell Binding Energy (E_K) of Various Elements

Element	Z	E_K (keV)
Aluminium	13	1.6
Calcium	20	4
Molybdenum	42	20
Iodine	53	33

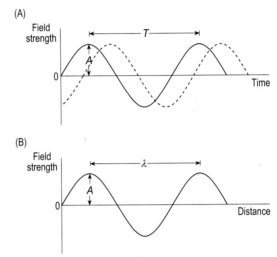

Fig. 1.6 Electromagnetic wave. Field strength versus (A) time and (B) distance.

TABLE 1.1 Some Fundamental Particles

	Relative Mass	Relative Charge	Symbol
Nucleons			
Neutron	1	0	n
Proton	1	+1	p
Extranuclear			
Electron	0.00054	−1	e$^-$, β$^-$
Other			
Positron	0.00054	+1	e$^+$, β$^+$
Alpha particle	4	+2	α

Combining particle and wave properties:

$$E = hf$$

where E = photon energy, h = Planck's constant, and f = frequency. Using $\lambda f = c$:

$$E = h/\lambda$$

showing that photon energy is inversely proportional to wavelength:

E (in keV) = 1.24/λ (in nm)
For example:
Blue light λ = 400 nm $E \approx$ 3 eV
X-/gamma rays λ = 0.1 nm E = 140 keV

Intensity

EM radiation irradiates all directions from a point source, with each 'ray' travelling in a straight line. Collimation of these rays allows for a beam in a given direction. The perpendicular cross-section of this beam allows for further characterisation. The main facets of a beam are photon fluence, energy fluence, beam intensity, and air kerma. Photon fluence (see Fig. 1.7a) is the number of photons that pass through a specified cross-section. Energy fluence is the sum energy of all photons passing this cross-section over a given time. Beam intensity indicates the energy

TABLE 1.3   Electromagnetic Spectrum

Radiation	Wavelength	Frequency	Energy
Radiowaves	1000–0.1 m	0.3–3000 MHz	0.001–10 µeV
Microwaves	100–1 mm	3–300 GHz	10–1000 µeV
Infrared	100–1 µm	3–300 THz	10–1000 MeV
Visible light	700–400 nm	430–750 THz	1.8–3 eV
Ultraviolet	400–10 nm	750–30,000 THz	1.8–100 eV
X- and gamma rays	1 nm–0.1 pm	3×10^5 to 3×10^9 THz	1 keV–10 MeV

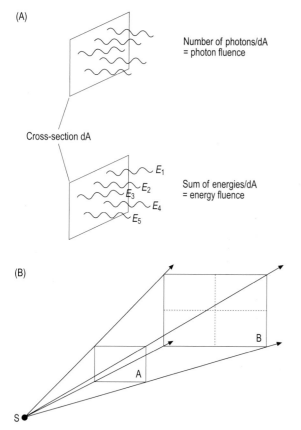

Fig. 1.7 (A) Photon fluence and energy fluence. (B) The inverse square law applying to a point source S.

fluence rate (W/mm²), including over time, but is difficult to measure in reality. Air kerma (kinetic energy released to matter) yields an indirect measurement of energy fluence.

Inverse square law (see Fig. 1.7b): The dimensions of a beam are proportional to distance. The area of a beam is proportional to the square of the distance from a point source. This relies on two assumptions:

1. Point source
2. There is no absorption or scatter between source and point of measurement

X-RAY TUBE AND X-RAY BEAM

X-rays are produced when fast-moving electrons undergo interaction with a metal target. The kinetic energy of the electrons is converted to X-rays (∼1%) and heat (∼99%).

X-ray Tube Overview
Production Overview

The cross-section of the X-ray tube anode/cathode is shown in Fig. 1.8. To generate electrons, the tungsten filament within the cathode is heated until incandescent. This enables thermionic emission to occur. This is the process through which a fraction of the free electrons can overcome the positive attraction of the metal anions. These free electrons are then focussed via the cup and attracted to the anode target (the degree of which is determined by the voltage). The electrons travel within a vacuum so that there is nothing else to interact with.

The electrical energy sources should have independently adjustable kilovoltage (kV) and milliamperage (mA) input settings.

The kV governs the accelerating voltage between anode and cathode (30–150 kV). It is determined by the waveform. High-frequency generators are used to maintain a near constant waveform (1% ripple). Previously varying types of rectification were used (see Fig. 1.9 and Box 1.2). The constant waveform has multiple advantages, including increased X-ray output and lower patient dose. The mA governs the tube current (energy and quantity of electrons flowing between anode and cathode). It is usually between 0.5 and 1000 mA.

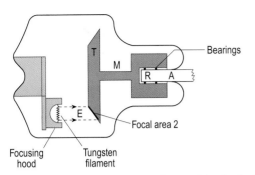

Fig. 1.8 Cross-section of the X-ray tube anode/cathode. T — rotating anode target disc; E — electron stream; M — Molybdenum stem; R — copper rotor.

(A)

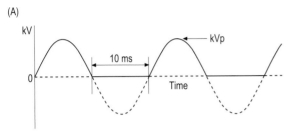

(B)

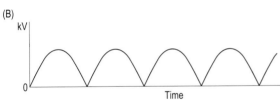

(C)

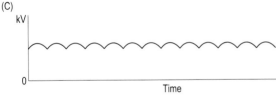

(D)

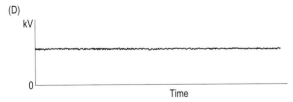

Fig. 1.9 Waveforms of high-voltage generators. (A) Single-phase, half wave—rectified, (B) single-phase, full wave—rectified, (C) three-phase, six-pulse, and (D) high-frequency generator.

Target Interactions

Electrons hit the target surface with kinetic energy (in keV) equivalent to the kV of the accelerating voltage. This yields one of two interactions:

Heat Production (~99%)

This is secondary to multiple small interactions and involves the outer electrons of target atoms.

X-ray Production (~1%)

This is secondary to interactions with:

Inner shell electrons: photoelectric effect and characteristic X-ray (see Fig. 1.10). A bombarding electron displaces an inner shell electron. This K-shell vacancy is filled by an L-shell electron (or, less likely, an M-shell electron). Characteristic photons are produced depending on which electrons fill the K-shell and the anode material. This line spectrum depends on the target atom (see Fig. 1.11 for tungsten).

- *Effective energy*: average energy (50%—60% of maximum)
- *Peak energy*: most common photon energy
  For tungsten:
- K-shell energy is 70 keV
- L-shell is 12 keV (Kα ~59 keV)
- M-shell is 2 keV (Kβ ~68 keV)

Field of the nucleus: the production of Bremsstrahlung (braking radiation), which accounts for 80% of produced X-rays (see Fig. 1.12). A bombarding electron passes through the electron shells and is deflected by the nucleus, losing some energy as radiation. This process yields a continuous spectrum of photon energies, dependent on tube voltage (see Fig. 1.11, dashed line).

Controlling the X-ray Spectrum

The modification of the following factors affects the X-ray spectrum (see Figs. 1.13—1.15):

kV

- Increased kV shifts the spectrum upwards and to the right
- Increased maximum and effective energy
- Increased total number of photons

mA

- Increased mA increases the quantity of photons only

BOX 1.1   SI Units

The SI system of units (le Système International d'Unités) for measurement uses a base set of quantities and units.

Mass	kilogram (kg)
Length	metre (m)
Time	second (s)
Amount of a substance	mole (mol)
Electric current	ampere (A)
Temperature	kelvin (K)
Luminous intensity	candela (cd)

All other units are derived from these. For example, the unit of energy is 1 kg m^2 s^{-2} and is given the special name joule (J), and the unit of power (watt, W) is equal to 1 J s^{-1}. The unit of electrical charge, the coulomb (C), is likewise derived from the base units and is the quantity of charge transported by a current of 1 A flowing for 1 s, 1 C = 1 As. The unit of electrical potential and electromotive force (EMF), the volt (V), is the EMF required for a charge of 1 C to acquire 1 J of energy, 1 V = 1 J C^{-1}.

In describing the energy of photons, it is common to use a derived unit that is not strictly defined in accordance with the SI convention that does not allow more or less arbitrary multipliers to be applied to the base units. The electronvolt (eV) is the energy acquired by an electron when it is accelerated through a potential difference of 1 V. As the charge of an electron is 1.6 × 10^{-19} C, the eV is equal to 1.6 × 10^{-19} J. It is convenient to use eV as a unit to describe the very small quantity of energy represented by a photon. In addition, it has direct relevance to the energy of X-rays generated by stopping electrons that have been accelerated to the kilovoltage (kV) applied across the X-ray tube. The maximum photon energy (keV$_{max}$) is simply numerically equal to the applied kV.

Other units derived from the SI base units will include the unit for absorbed dose, gray (Gy, 1 Gy = 1 J kg^{-1}), and the unit of activity, becquerel (Bq, 1 Bq = 1 s^{-1}).

Units may also have multiplying factors that can be used conveniently to describe very large or small amounts of any quantity. These are as follows:

pico (p)	10^{-12}
nano (n)	10^{-9}
micro (μ)	10^{-6}
milli (m)	10^{-3}
kilo (k)	10^{3}
mega (M)	10^{6}
giga (G)	10^{9}
tera (T)	10^{12}

BOX 1.2   X-Ray Waveform

The function of the X-ray generator is to produce a high voltage to be applied between the anode and cathode. High voltage can be produced from a low voltage, alternating current (AC) supply (the mains) using a transformer to give the waveform in Fig. 1.9a. The time between peaks is 20 ms for the 50 Hz mains frequency used in the UK. Because electrons are generated in the filament, the tube current can flow from the filament to the target only during the positive phase of the kilovoltage (kV) cycle. This type of generator is described as *single-phase, self-rectified*. It is commonly used in dental radiography equipment.

Rectification is the process of converting the negative part of the waveform into a positive kV and, in its simplest form, converts the standard waveform into the pulsating direct current (DC) waveform as shown in Fig. 1.9b; *full wave—rectified, single-phase*. More complex circuitry using all three phases of the mains supply may be used to produce near constant potential with a small ripple, as shown in Fig. 1.9c. The three-phase generator has six or 12 pulses per cycle and an associated ripple theoretically equal to 13% and 4%, respectively.

Full wave—rectified and three-phase generators are no longer manufactured. Modern X-ray equipment uses high-frequency (HF) generators in which the mains is converted to HF AC (1 kHz or higher), and this can be converted to a steady high-voltage DC supply with no more than 1% ripple (Fig. 1.9d). HF generators are particularly compact and stable.

The anode–cathode voltage is often stated in terms of its peak value (kVp), although the terminology kV is more common in modern generators.

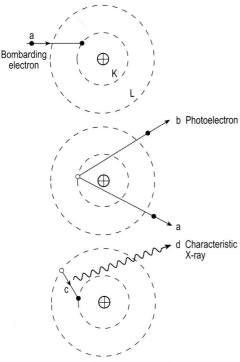

Fig. 1.10 Production of characteristic radiation.

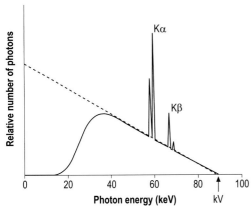

Fig. 1.11 An X-ray spectrum for tungsten.

Filtration

- Moves the continuous spectrum to the right
- Increases minimum and effective energy
- Reduces the total number of photons
- Increases the receptor:skin ratio (exit dose:entry dose)

Waveform

- Uniform constant current allows for an increased quantity of photons and effective energy

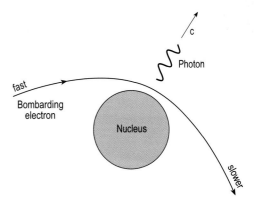

Fig. 1.12 Production of Bremsstrahlung.

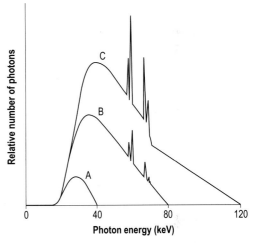

Fig. 1.13 Effect of tube kilovoltage (kV) on X-ray spectra for three tube potentials. A = 40kV, B = 80kV, C = 120kV.

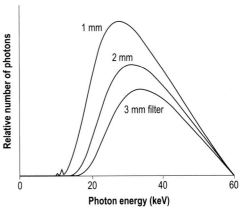

Fig. 1.14 Effect of increasing aluminium filtration on the X-ray spectrum.

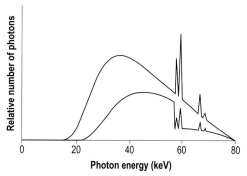

Relative number of photons

Photon energy (keV)

Fig. 1.15 Effect of a 0.1 mm erbium filter on the spectrum at 80 kV compared with the same beam filtered by 2.5 mm Al.

Atomic Number of Target

- Varies the amount of Bremsstrahlung and energy of characteristic photons

FILTRATION

Filtration involves the removal of lower-energy photons before they reach the patient. Lower-energy photons mostly contribute to the dose and have little impact on image formation.

The total filtration for a system is equivalent to the sum of inherent and additional filtration. For general radiology, this is 2.5 mm aluminium equivalent and removes X-rays <20 keV.

Inherent filtration in the system, equivalent to 1 mm aluminium. This is contributed by the target material itself (e.g. anode heel effect (see Ch. 3)) and the X-ray tube housing window.

Additional filtration from a flat sheet placed between tube and patient, usually composed of aluminium.

The choice of filter material is determined by atomic number (Z). This needs to be high enough to make the process of photoelectric absorption predominant. Aluminium ($Z = 13$, $E_K = 1.6$ keV) is most common.

The effects of filtration are demonstrated in Fig. 1.14. Filtration attenuates lower-energy X-rays more than higher-energy X-rays:

- Increases the half-value layer (HVL)/penetrating power
- Reduces intensity
- Reduces skin dose

Increasing the filtration has the following effects:

- Shrinks the overall continuous X-ray spectrum
- Right-shifts the X-ray spectrum
- Increases the minimum and effective photon energies
- Reduces overall output of X-rays
- Can increase the required exposure time

Specific filters include:

- The K-edge filter is used extensively in mammography. It removes both high- and low-energy X-rays (see Fig. 1.15)
- The wedge filter is shaped to create a more uniform exposure across a radiograph

MATTER INTERACTIONS

X-rays/Gamma Rays

There are different possible outcomes for each photon as it travels through matter (see Fig. 1.16):

Transmission — Photon passes through unaffected as primary radiation and is the principal photon in X-ray image formation

Absorption — Photon transfers all energy to the matter, and the photon disappears

Scatter — Diverted in a new direction with or without the loss of energy, as secondary radiation

Each of these outcomes is a stochastic process governed by the statistical laws of chance. The outcome of any given photon is impossible to predict. The overall outcome of a beam with a large number of photons can be accurately predicted.

Attenuation

There are fewer photons present in a beam after it has passed through material than when it entered due to absorption and scatter. Overall, this process is called attenuation. Attenuation of a narrow, monoenergetic beam of X-rays is governed by:

$$I = I_0 e^{-\mu d}$$

where I = intensity, I_0 = incident X-ray intensity, μ = linear attenuation coefficient (see below), and d = thickness of the material (see Fig. 1.17).

The HVL is the thickness of a given material that will halve the intensity of a narrow beam of X-radiation (dashed lines in Fig. 1.17). The reduction in intensity is governed by 2^x (where x is the number of HVLs). Three HVLs would equate to $2^3 = 8$; 10 HVLs would equate to $2^{10} = 1024$.

The linear attenuation coefficient (μ in cm^{-1}) is specific to each material. It quantifies attenuating properties and indicates the probability of a photon interacting in a given material.

$$\mu = \ln2/HVL$$

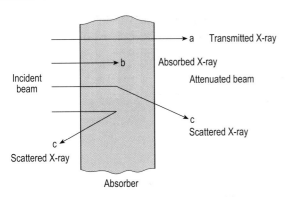

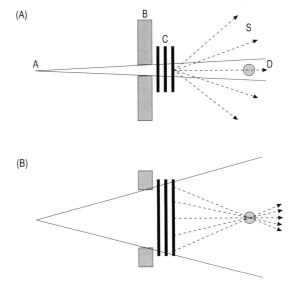

Fig. 1.16 Interaction of X- or gamma rays with matter.

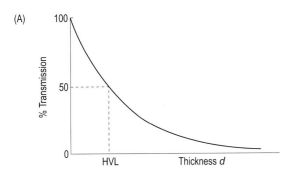

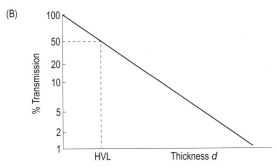

Fig. 1.17 Exponential attenuation, HVLs. (A) Linear scale and (B) logarithmic scale. HVL, half-value layer.

Fig. 1.18 (A) A narrow beam is used for the measurement of the half-value layer. (B) Transmission of a wide beam.

The width of the beam impacts upon the attenuation, with there being an increased contribution of scatter on a detector with a wider beam (see Fig. 1.18). The measured HVL, in this case, would be increased.

Heterogeneous Beam Attenuation

X-ray tubes produce polyenergetic beams (rather than monoenergetic). Lower-energy photons are removed proportionally more than high-energy photons, yielding beam hardening. The more a beam passes through a material, the less heterogeneous it becomes, with an increased proportion of higher-energy photons. The second HVL is larger than the first HVL as the hardened beam has more high-energy photons. The exponential attenuation curve can still be applied to produce approximate HVL thicknesses.

Compton Effect

X-ray interaction with a loosely bound or free electron, yielding inelastic/non-coherent scattering is known as Compton effect. The electron absorbs some of the photon energy as kinetic energy (see Fig. 1.19). The recoil electron is projected forwards or sideways with higher energy. There is scatter of the incident photon in a new direction with reduced energy. The scatter angle θ between the incident and scattered photon determines energy transfer (in the diagnostic energy range, $\leq 20\%$ is transferred to an electron). As θ increases:

Mass attenuation coefficient (MAC) indicates the rate of energy loss through an area of material and is independent of density:

$$MAC = \mu/\rho$$

HVL decreases / LAC increases:
- Increased density of material
- Increased atomic number of material
- Decreased incident photon energy

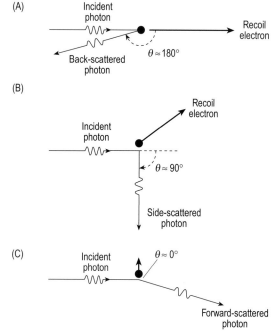

(A)

(B)

(C)

Fig. 1.19 Compton scattering by a free electron.

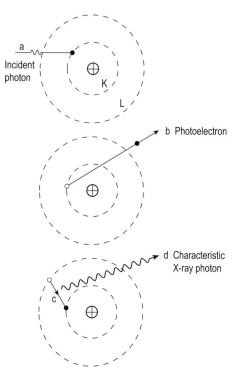

Fig. 1.20 Photoelectric absorption.

- Increased kinetic energy imparted to the recoil electron (increased range)
- Decreased energy of the scattered photon (with increased wavelength)

The Compton process is governed by $\sigma = \rho/E$ and contributes to the linear attenuation coefficient (μ), where σ = Compton linear attenuation coefficient, ρ = physical density, and E = electron density. This is independent of Z. The value is approximately $1/E$ for diagnostic radiology energy levels.

Photoelectric Effect

An incident X-/gamma ray photon collides with a bound K-shell electron allowing ejection of the electron (photoelectron); see Fig. 1.20. The energy of the incident photon is completely absorbed in this process.

Kinetic energy of electron = photon energy – E_k

Part of the energy is required to release the energy from the atom (binding energy, E_k). Sometimes the photon interacts with an electron in the L-shell with binding energy E_L.

Each ejected photoelectron leaves a hole in the electron shell that is filled by a higher-energy level electron, releasing characteristic radiation. This characteristic radiation is low energy and is absorbed immediately with the release of an Auger electron (very low energy).

Photoelectric absorption in low atomic number material (e.g. human tissue) yields complete absorption of incident photon energy.

$$\mu = \sigma + \tau$$

where σ = Compton linear attenuation coefficient and τ = photoelectric linear attenuation coefficient.

$$\tau \propto \rho Z^3 / E^3$$

where ρ = density; Z = atomic number and E = incident photon energy.

The probability of photoelectric absorption decreases with increased incident photon energy ($1/E^3$) and increases with the increased atomic number of the material (Z^3); see Fig. 1.21.

Absorption edges indicate the sudden increase in probability of photoelectric absorption as incident photon energy reaches K/L/M-shell binding energies (see Fig. 1.11).

Different interactions predominate over different ranges of photon energies (see Fig. 1.22). In most radiology applications, photon energies are <1 MeV, so only photoelectric and Compton effects are considered.

Secondary Electrons

These encompass recoil electrons and photoelectrons. These are both directly ionising and tend to interact with the outer shells of atoms:
- Excite the atom — 3 eV
- Ionise the atom — 10 eV
- Electron loses ~34 eV per ion pair formed

The range of a secondary electron is the distance it can travel before losing its initial excitation energy and is inversely proportional to the density of the material. The excitations and ionisations of secondary electrons can cause a number of effects:

- Ionisation of air/gas makes them electrically conducting
- Ionisation of atoms in cells causes biological damage
- Photographic effect
- Blackening of silver and bromine in photographic film
- Plain film radiography
- Excitation of phosphors allows for luminescence/fluorescence
- Excitation allows increased molecular motion causing heating

Charged Particles

This section entails a brief overview of some of the interactions of charged particles (other than electrons) with matter. The more detailed explanations are very equation heavy and beyond the scope of this book, but an overview of how charged particles interact is important. Charged particles behave differently from photons due to mass and charge. Charged particles have a surrounding electrostatic field (coulomb field). Interactions with matter yield the concept of stopping power:
- Collision — energy deposited locally
- Radiative — energy dispersed as photons

Charged particles have a range, an ultimate depth within matter (unlike photons which undergo exponential decay). The range is dependent upon the initial energy and particle type (see Fig. 1.23).

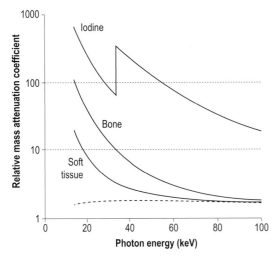

Fig. 1.21 Mass attenuation coefficients as a function of energy. Photoelectric effect (solid lines) for soft tissue, bone and iodine, and Compton effect (dashed line) averaged for all tissues.

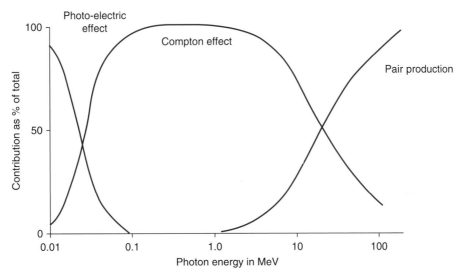

Fig. 1.22 Relative dominance of different matter interactions dependent on photon energy.

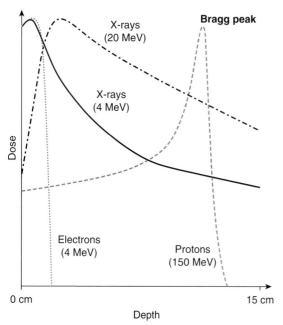

Fig. 1.23 Bragg curve.

Some of the main types of interactions are:
- Soft collisions:
  - Atom can be excited or ionised (valence shell electron ejected)
  - Most probable type
- Hard collisions:
  - Interaction with an individual electron that gets ejected as a delta ray
  - Characteristic X-ray or Auger electron also produced
- Nuclear field interaction:
  - Deflection (almost elastic scattering)
  - Bremsstrahlung
  Heavy particle nuclear interactions:
- Inelastic
- Expulsion of nucleons (intranuclear cascade)
- Deposition of energy to the nucleus causing excitation and subsequent evaporation of particles and gamma rays

LUMINESCENCE

Luminescence is the process through which a material absorbs energy and then re-emits this energy in the form of visible photons. This occurs in relatively cool materials, differing from incandescence (e.g. burning wood). In radiology, we are concerned with photoluminescence (the energy source is EM radiation).

Luminescence depends on the electron shells present in a molecule. In a stable molecule, the valence electron shell is completely filled to facilitate stability. The next highest electron shell, which is empty at ground state, is called the conduction band. When energy is deposited in the material, the valence shell electrons excite and move into the conduction band. Within the conduction band, there are multiple energy states for the excited electron to occupy; the electron can also move freely within the material whole. As the excited electron loses some energy through non-radiative decay (vibrational energy or heat), it drops between the individual layers of the conduction band. As the excited electron drops from the valence shell, the energy is released as a photon, often of lower energy and longer wavelength than the incident EM radiation (see Fig. 1.24).

Fluorescence involves the emission of the photon(s) nearly instantaneously (time scale 10^{-10} to 10^{-7} s).

Phosphorescence involves delayed emission of the photon(s). This is facilitated by the introduction of impurities in compounds. These impurities are additional elements that can form part of the main material but have differing energy shell levels (referred to as electron traps). To reach one of these electron traps, the excited electron first loses some energy through intersystem crossing (to reach the impurity element). Then the electron can drop into an electron trap [Further reading: triplet state]. To return from here to the native valence shell, the energy shell is now considered 'forbidden' due to the conservation of angular momentum. Even though transitions from the electron trap to the valence energy are forbidden, they still occur, just at a much slower rate than fluorescence, hence the time delay to phosphorescence (10^{-6} to 10 s). Some electron traps are stable and do not facilitate transition without further energy input.

Thermoluminescence enables the transition of the electrons and hence the emission of photons via heating. In photostimulable luminescence, the irradiated phosphor is exposed to light. If the incident photon is of the same energy as the photon resulting from fluorescence, this is termed resonance excitation. This only occurs when monochromatic light is used and yields a luminescence efficiency of 100%. The majority of luminescence is not at 100% (solid phosphors at ~20%, electroluminescence at ~10%). The intensity of the light emitted by phosphorescence is proportional to the incident energy absorbed. In radiology, this is proportional to the intensity of the radiation beam itself.

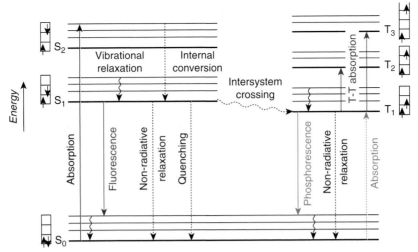

Fig. 1.24 Jablonski diagram. An electron at an energy level/shell of S0 is excited to the state S1/2. It loses some energy through vibrational relaxation until the lowest state of S1/2 is reached. At this point, it fluoresces back to S0 with the release of a photon of energy, *hv*. It can instead undergo intersystem crossing into a different excited state, T_1. If the electron directly returns to S0 from this state via photon release, this is termed phosphorescence.

RADIOACTIVITY

Stable Nuclei

Nuclides are atoms with specific numbers of protons and neutrons in their nucleus. There are over 300 naturally occurring nuclides on earth, of which around 250 are stable, and around 90 are unstable (radioactive). The stable nuclei of the lighter elements contain approximately equal numbers of protons and neutrons, except hydrogen, which has only a single proton in its nucleus. Nuclei heavier than calcium-40 (^{40}Ca) have a greater proportion of neutrons to maintain the optimal spacing arrangement for the interactions of the strong nuclear force within the nucleus.

Isotopes

Nuclides containing the same number of protons and different numbers of neutrons are *isotopes* of an element. These will have the same atomic number and chemical properties but will have different atomic mass numbers, density, and other physical properties.

For example, carbon has four isotopes, the nuclei of which all contain six protons. Three occur naturally: the stable isotopes carbon-12 (^{12}C), with six neutrons, and carbon-13 (^{13}C), with seven neutrons, and the unstable, radioactive isotope carbon-14 (^{14}C). This has a neutron excess, having eight neutrons. The final isotope carbon-11 (^{11}C) is also unstable and radioactive and can only be produced artificially. It is neutron deficient, having only five neutrons.

Radionuclides

Radionuclides have an unstable configuration of protons and neutrons in their nucleus, either deficit or excess, and undergo nuclear transformations (also called decay) to alter the balance between these. This is achieved by the emission of any combination of alpha, beta, and gamma radiation, and the process will continue until the nucleus reaches a stable configuration.

Radionuclide Production

There are three main methods of production of the radionuclides used in medical imaging. These are using
- A cyclotron
- A nuclear reactor
- A radionuclide generator

Cyclotron

Cyclotrons produce radionuclides by bombarding stable nuclei with highly energetic charged particles, typically protons. These force neutrons out of the target nuclei, leaving these in an unstable configuration with a neutron deficit. In this case, the mass number is unchanged, but the atomic number is increased by one, meaning a change to a new element.

The most common example is the production of fluorine-18 (^{18}F) which is used in positron emission tomography (PET).

$$^{18}O + p \rightarrow ^{18}F + n$$

Oxygen-18 undergoes proton bombardment and produces the required fluorine-18. The resulting neutron flux complicates the shielding requirements for these facilities. There is a range of minicyclotrons which have been developed for the on-site generation of short-lived radionuclides for PET. These are generally sited at, or close to, the hospitals that require the radionuclides, although the high capital costs of these facilities, at least partly due to the complex shielding requirements, mean that many hospital sites rely upon commercial suppliers rather than having their own facility.

The radionuclides produced in cyclotrons can be obtained at high purities as they can be separated from the original stable nuclides relatively simply due to their different chemical properties, which result from their differing atomic numbers.

Nuclear Reactor

There are two methods of radionuclide production which can be achieved using reactors.

The simplest is the extraction of fission products from the spent fuel rods, which can be achieved to high purities due to their different chemical forms. The commonest fission product is iodine-131 (^{131}I) which is used for therapeutic treatments.

$$^{238}U \rightarrow ^{131}I + \text{other fission products}$$

The second method is the bombardment of stable nuclei by neutrons from the high neutron flux prevalent in reactor cores. This creates unstable radionuclides with a neutron excess. The most common radionuclide produced by this method is molybdenum-99 (^{99}Mo), which is used in the production of technetium-99m (^{99}Tc^m).

$$^{98}Mo + n \rightarrow ^{99}Mo$$

The similar chemical properties of the different forms of molybdenum make separation of these problematic, and it is difficult to obtain very high purity samples.

Radionuclide Generator

These are generally used to produce shorter-lived radionuclides which cannot be produced in a cyclotron but can be produced from the decay of a longer-lived radionuclide. The longer-lived radionuclides are referred to as *parent* radionuclides, and the shorter-lived products are known as *daughter* radionuclides. Commonly available daughter products include ^{99m}Tc from a ^{99}Mo (^{99}Tc^m/^{99}Mo) generator and krypton-81m (^{81}Kr^m) from a rubidium-81 (^{81}Kr^m/^{81}Rb) generator.

New Production Developments

The nuclear reactors used for radionuclide production are not the power generation reactors commonly found around the world but are smaller research reactors which are less common. Many of these are approaching, or have already passed, their planned operating lifetimes and require higher maintenance requirements to keep them operational. In recent years, this has led to a number of unplanned shutdowns and failures of different facilities, resulting in major disruption to the global supply of ^{99}Mo and consequent impacts on nuclear medicine departments worldwide. For this reason, considerable investment has been made to develop alternative methods of production of ^{99}Mo or methods of direct production of ^{99}Tc^m.

One method under development is the use of neutron generators to bombard ^{98}Mo for the production of ^{99}Mo. The neutron generators are often based around small linear particle accelerators, which fuse isotopes of hydrogen to produce the neutrons.

Another approach is the direct production of ^{99}Tc^m using cyclotrons. Unfortunately, the power requirements needed to achieve this precludes the use of the common medical cyclotrons and requires specialist facilities to achieve this. Another drawback of this approach is the higher levels of contaminants in the ^{99}Tc^m produced, as this tends to contain numerous additional radioisotopes of technetium. This increases the radiation dose to the patient from a specific administered dose of ^{99}Tc^m and can affect the labelling efficiency of pharmaceutical kits for the production of radiopharmaceuticals.

There have also been a small number of new research reactors commissioned around the world, which have increased the capacity for irradiation of molybdenum and, to some extent, alleviated the immediate problem. One example of this is the Open Pool Australian Light-water reactor in the southern suburbs of Sydney, Australia.

RADIOACTIVE DECAY

The decay (or transformation) method of a particular radionuclide depends on the balance of protons and neutrons within its nucleus. Each radionuclide emits a unique combination of alpha, beta, and gamma radiations with energies characteristic of that radionuclide.

Radionuclides with a Neutron Excess

Radionuclides with too many neutrons for stability decay by **beta** decay (sometimes referred to as beta minus decay (β^- decay) to differentiate it from positron (β^+ decay). In beta decay, a neutron is converted into a proton and an electron. The electron is emitted from the nucleus in the form of a beta particle.

$$n \rightarrow p + \beta^-$$

The daughter nuclide thus has the same mass number as the parent, with the atomic number increased by 1.

$$^A_Z\text{Parent} \rightarrow\ ^A_{Z+1}\text{Daughter} + \beta^-$$

Generally, the daughter nucleus is produced in an excess energy state and returns immediately to its ground, or minimum energy, state by releasing a number of gamma photons.

Isomeric Transition

Metastable radionuclides decay by isomeric transition. These do not return to their ground state instantaneously but exist for longer periods before decaying to the ground state. The energy difference between the excited and ground states is emitted as gamma radiation. The mass number and atomic number are unchanged by isomeric transitions so that the parent and daughter radionuclides are identical in all respects other than their energy states and half-lives. The parent and daughter radionuclides are referred to as *isomers*.

The most widely known metastable radionuclide is $^{99}\text{Tc}^m$, which decays to technetium-99 (^{99}Tc) with the emission of 140 keV gamma rays. This pure gamma emission makes $^{99}\text{Tc}^m$ ideally suited as an imaging radionuclide as all the emitted radiation contributes to the formation of a useable image, which is not the case where there are particulate emissions of beta or alpha particles.

The decay scheme for $^{99}\text{Tc}^m$ can then be written as:

$$^{99}_{42}\text{Mo} \xrightarrow{\beta^-\ \gamma}\ ^{99}_{43}\text{Tc}^m \xrightarrow{\gamma}\ ^{99}_{43}Tc \xrightarrow{\beta^-\ \gamma}\ ^{99}_{44}\text{Ru}$$

where ruthenium-99 is the stable nuclide at the end of the decay chain.

Beta Emission

The spectrum of beta-emitting radionuclides does not exhibit the characteristic photopeak(s) of gamma-emitting radionuclides but instead covers a continuous spectrum up to a maximum value, E_{max}, which is characteristic of the radionuclide. The average energy of the beta particles is approximately $E_{max}/3$. Irrespective of their charge, when the moving electrons of beta emissions travel through a substance, they will interact with the outer shell electrons of adjacent atoms, causing ionisation. This leads the track of the beta particles to be dotted with ion pairs.

The beta particle will lose energy during these interactions until it has depleted its initial energy, at which point it reaches the end of its range. The range depends upon the initial energy of the beta particle and the density of the material through which it is travelling. Typically, this is a few millimetres in tissue.

Radionuclides with a Neutron Deficit

These can also be described as having a proton excess, which can be resolved by the conversion of a proton into a neutron and a positive electron. This is released from the nucleus as a high-energy, positive beta particle, commonly referred to as a *positron*. Positrons are a type of antimatter. Antimatter particles have an opposite charge to their matching particle. Positrons are the antimatter equivalent of electrons.

$$p \rightarrow n + \beta^+$$

The atomic number thus reduces by one, and the mass number stays the same. As with negative beta decay, the daughter nucleus may be left in an excited state, releasing gamma energy until the ground state is reached.

An alternative means of decay for nuclei with a proton excess is the capture of an inner (K) shell electron, facilitating the conversion of a proton into a neutron. This is known as *electron capture* and leads to outer shell electrons cascading down to fill the vacancy in the K-shell, with the emission of characteristic X-rays. If left in an excited state, the daughter nucleus may also emit gamma rays.

$$p + e^- \rightarrow n$$

Again, the atomic number reduces by one, and the mass number is unchanged. A commonly found example in nuclear medicine is iodine-123 (^{123}I) which decays purely by electron capture with the emission of 160 keV gamma and 28 keV X-rays.

Positron Emitters

A positron emitted by a neutron deficient nucleus is antimatter, the antiparticle of a negative electron, and therefore exists for only a very short time before interacting with a free electron. The matter—antimatter particles cannot coexist, and both disappear, with their mass being converted to energy. From Einstein's famous equation $E = mc^2$, it is relatively straightforward to calculate that the mass of a positron has an energy equivalence of 511 keV. A positron—electron pair has an energy equivalence of 1.02 MeV, and this is the threshold energy difference between parent and daughter nuclear energy levels for radionuclides to be able to decay by positron emission. The energy is emitted in the form of two 511 keV gamma rays travelling collinearly in opposite directions. This 511 keV gamma radiation, sometimes known as annihilation radiation, is the basis of PET image formation.

Internal Conversion

Some radionuclides undergo *internal conversion* where the emitted gamma rays from the nucleus are absorbed by K-shell electrons which are then ejected from the atom via the photoelectric effect. This results in the emission of characteristic X-rays and photoelectrons, which make these radionuclides generally unsuitable for imaging as the X-rays are of insufficient energy to escape the body and only contribute unnecessary radiation dose to the patient.

Processes of Radioactive Decay

Radioactive decay is a random process which obeys Poisson statistics. This means that it is impossible to determine when any particular unstable nucleus will disintegrate, but when there are large numbers of nuclei, the rate at which they will decay is predictable.

The amount of radioactive decay is known as radioactivity or simply activity. The activity of a radionuclide is the number of nuclear transformations per second. It may also be referred to as the number of disintegrations per

second or **becquerels** (Bq). The becquerel is the SI unit of activity, but in imaging, we generally use megabecquerels (1 MBq = 10^6 Bq) and gigabecquerels (1 GBq = 10^9 Bq).

Once a nucleus has decayed, then it cannot do it again. Thus, the number of atoms available to decay continuously decreases with time. The time taken to decay depends on the instability of the radionuclide and is characterised by its **half-life.**

After one half-life ($t_{1/2}$), the activity is reduced to one half of its original value. After n half-lives, the activity will have been reduced by a factor of 2^n. Mathematically radioactive decay is an exponential process, with the radioactivity of a sample being proportional to the number of radioactive atoms present.

For a given element, the nucleus has the same probability of decaying per second, λ. So if we have N atoms, the number of decays per second, i.e. the activity:

$$A = -\lambda N$$

Thus, we can write mathematically:

$$N = N_0 e^{-\lambda t}$$

where N_0 is the number of parent nuclei at time $t = 0$, N is the number of undecayed nuclei t seconds later and λ is the probability of decay or decay constant. This is related to the half-life ($t_{1/2}$) by the formula:

$$\lambda = \ln 2 / t_{1/2} = 0.693 / t_{1/2}$$

The activity can be seen to also follow an exponential relationship and can be written as:

$$A = A_0 e^{-\lambda t}$$

This can be plotted graphically, as seen in Fig. 1.25, using linear axes, which demonstrates the characteristic exponential curve shape. This also clearly demonstrates that the activity never falls to zero.

If the activity is instead plotted on a logarithmic scale (see Fig. 1.26), the resultant decay curve is a straight line of slope $-\lambda$ and with an intercept of $\ln A_0$.

Curves of this form make it comparatively straightforward to determine how long radioactive waste must be stored before it can be safely disposed of. These can also be used to calculate the amount of activity that must be prepared to have a particular amount available a given number of hours later.

The correct definition for the half-life which we have been describing here is the physical half-life, t_{phys}, which is

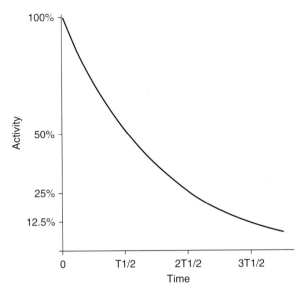

Fig. 1.25 Graph of the total radioactivity of a sample during decay using linear axes.

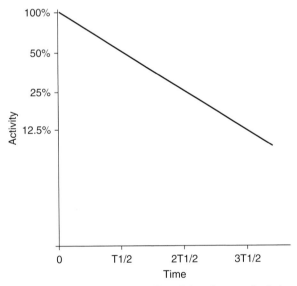

Fig. 1.26 Graph of the total radioactivity of a sample during decay using log-linear axes.

an immutable property of the radionuclide. These can range from fractions of a second to trillions of years. Bismuth-209 has a physical half-life more than a billion times greater than the current age of the universe.

From an imaging point of view, we also need to consider the physiological clearance of the pharmaceutical compound to which any radionuclide has been joined,

which is known as labelling. This determines the clearance of the pharmaceutical from the body tissues and can again be described using an exponential model. As such, it also has a half-life to define the clearance rate, and this is known as the biological half-life, t_{biol}.

In the body, the clearance of any combination of a pharmaceutical and a radionuclide is determined by the combined effects of the radioactive decay and the physiological clearance. This will be shorter than the physical or biological half-lives as both occur simultaneously. It will also vary subtly amongst any population group as the physiological processes are unique to each individual and may be affected by any current pathology.

This combined clearance can be said to be occurring with a half-life known as the effective half-live, t_{eff}. This is defined mathematically as:

$$1 / t_{eff} = 1 / t_{phys} + 1 / t_{biol}$$

Characteristics of an Ideal Radionuclide

Any radionuclide being considered for use in imaging should have as many as possible of a group of desirable properties which allow optimisation of imaging parameters whilst minimising radiation exposure to the patient and staff. These are:

- A physical half-life which is similar in length to the total time of the imaging examination from the preparation of the product to the end of the imaging. This is generally a few hours
- Emission of gamma rays only, with no particulate emissions or low-energy gamma and X-rays, as these only contribute dose to the patient with no imaging benefit. This indicates that decay by isomeric transition or electron capture are preferable
- Emission of monoenergetic gamma rays as this allows simpler exclusion of scattered radiation
- Gamma rays with sufficient energy to easily leave the patient's body but low enough to be easily detected by the imaging system. The optimal energy is around 150 keV, but energies between 50–400 keV can be tolerated
- Decay to a stable daughter product or one with a half-life which is sufficiently longer than the average human lifespan
- Should be chemically versatile to allow simple labelling to any required pharmaceutical with no significant detriment to its biological behaviour
- Should be easily available, ideally with a means of production on the site of the imaging facility

The radionuclide that comes closest to these ideal parameters and is the most commonly used in nuclear medicine is $^{99}Tc^m$. This decays by isomeric transition with a 6 hours half-life and produces monoenergetic 140 keV gamma rays. It can be produced on-site using a ^{99}Mo generator and, as a transition metal, is chemically versatile.

RADIOPHARMACEUTICALS

The combination of radionuclides labelled with pharmaceutical preparations used as diagnostic or therapeutic agents are known as radiopharmaceuticals. If we can find a pharmaceutical that is trapped in or handled by a particular organ of interest, we can image any organ system in the body.

The ideal radiopharmaceutical should have the following properties:

- Be specific to the pathology of interest, i.e. localise predominantly in the organ system of interest
- Have a short biological half-life, such that the majority is excreted from the body shortly after the conclusion of the imaging
- Be non-toxic or of very low toxicity
- Be stable both *in vitro* and *in vivo*
- Be readily available and economic

Preparation of Radiopharmaceuticals

There are three commonly used basic methods of production of radiopharmaceuticals:

- Substitution of a stable nuclide with a radionuclide
- Addition of a radionuclide to a chemical compound
- Incorporation of a radionuclide onto autologous blood cells

Substitution of a Stable Nuclide

This is used to image processes involving biologically useful elements where the stable form can be replaced by a radionuclide of suitable characteristics. The most common example is the use of ^{123}I to image the thyroid. In practice, all radiopharmaceuticals produced by this method are prepared by a commercial manufacturer and distributed to the user in sterile vials with stated activity, volume, and reference time.

Addition to a Chemical Compound

This is the method used for the production of most radiopharmaceuticals in nuclear medicine departments. $^{99}Tc^m$ labelled radiopharmaceuticals are prepared on a daily basis in a radiopharmacy facility. This may be on the hospital site or, in larger urban centres, a central facility

may transport the prepared products out to the different hospital sites.

The unlabelled pharmaceutical material and required chemicals are generally supplied as a freeze-dried powder in a sterile vial. These are often known as radiopharmaceutical *kits*. The user adds the required activity of sterile eluate (sodium pertechnetate, $NaTcO_4$) from the $^{99}Tc^m$ generator to the kit vial. Usually, labelling is completed in a few minutes with little intervention except agitation to ensure mixing. Further steps, such as immersion in a boiling water bath for a short period, are required for some preparations.

Blood Cell Labelling

Autologous blood cell labelling is one of the most complex procedures undertaken in radiopharmacies. The patient's blood is centrifuged to separate the component cells of the blood then the required cells can be extracted for labelling. White blood cells and platelets are labelled *in vitro* and then resuspended in the extracted plasma or a saline solution for injection back into the patient. *In vitro* labelling of cells must be performed in separate facilities from those used for general radiopharmaceutical production due to the high level of sterility required and the risk of cross-infection.

Red blood cells can be labelled *in vitro,* but for imaging purposes using $^{99}Tc^m$ are generally labelled *in vivo* by prior injection of a reducing agent, stannous chloride ($SnCl_2$). This adheres to the surface of the red cells, and when a subsequent injection of sodium pertechnetate is administered, the pertechnetate ion adheres strongly to the stannous ion. This provides a simple method of cell labelling with a very high labelling efficiency, generally over 95%.

Advantages of Kit Preparation

The advantages of kit preparation of radiopharmaceuticals which ensures it is the most commonly used method are:

- Rapid and easy preparation of the product
- Low radiation hazard to the operator as handling time is minimised
- Radiopharmaceutical product is stable, sterile, and pyrogen-free
- Radiopharmaceutical product is reproducible and reliable
- The unlabelled kit material has a long shelf life, generally a few months, which simplifies stock control and allows for the use of regular standing orders
- The kits are generally readily available and economical to procure as there is a robust market with sufficient competition to ensure competitive pricing

Most radiopharmaceuticals are administered by injection (usually intravenous) and therefore must be sterile. This does not apply to radiopharmaceuticals that are administered orally or by inhalation. The radiopharmaceutical may be diluted with saline in the preparation vial to give an appropriate concentration.

The prepared radiopharmaceutical with the appropriate activity may be dispensed into sterile syringes for patient administration or decanted into further sterile vials, which are sent to the hospital nuclear medicine department. The required volume can then be drawn up from the vial into a syringe just prior to injection to ensure the correct activity is administered. This method gives greater flexibility than the direct distribution of pre-prepared syringes as the department can easily adjust if the patient arrives early or late. Once labelled, radiopharmaceuticals generally have a limited shelf life of typically 4–8 hours, or more practically, the end of the working day on the day of production.

Radiopharmaceuticals for injection must be produced in a sterile, pyrogen-free environment. The required standards of air cleanliness for the preparation of sterile products are classified as Grades A, B, C, and D under the Good Manufacturing Practice[1] (GMP) guidelines. All aseptic operations should be in a workstation with a controlled work environment conforming to GMP Grade A. This can be provided by a laminar flow cabinet in a cleanroom or an isolator with a filtered air supply. If using a laminar flow cabinet, the cleanroom must conform to at least Grade B standard. Blood cell labelling must be conducted in a laminar flow cabinet or isolator in a separate room from other radiopharmaceutical production.

Laminar flow cabinets are similar to fume hoods but of considerably higher performance and specification. The work area is flushed with a nonturbulent, unidirectional downflow of filtered high-efficiency particulate air, which can be recycled. Cleanrooms are positively pressurised, environmentally controlled workrooms, where entry and egress are through a cascading, positively pressurised three-stage changing area. Isolators have integral lead shielding and allow the operator to manipulate materials within via an integrated glove system. They are generally negatively pressurised to mitigate against leaks and provide very high rates of air exchange.

Quality Control

All radiopharmaceutical production must be compliant with the appropriate local legislation, which in the UK includes the Medicines Act[2] and IRR[3] and requires appropriate permissions from the MHRA. A major part of all legislation and licencing is the maintenance of adequate quality control. Therefore, all radiopharmaceuticals produced undergo a number of quality checks which include:

Radionuclide Activity

This is to ensure that the correct, required amount of activity is being produced and is measured using an air ionisation chamber. These are often known as radionuclide or dose calibrators. Syringes or vials can be measured by sitting them in a holder which drops into the well of the calibrator. An electric current is generated by the ionisation of the air in the chamber, which is proportional to the radioactivity of the selected radionuclide. Preset buttons are generally available for common radionuclides, or bespoke radionuclides can be measured if the correct calibration value is known. The measured activity is indicated on a digital display, usually in megabecquerels, and some now have touchscreen displays to minimise space requirements.

Radionuclide Purity

This test measures the proportion of the radioactivity present, which is in the stated radionuclide form. A possible contaminant in $^{99}Tc^m$ radiopharmaceuticals is ^{99}Mo from the generator column if this has washed off during elution of the generator. Testing should be carried out daily for molybdenum breakthrough by placing the freshly eluted sodium pertechnetate solution vial in a 6-mm thick lead container and measuring the ionisation current in the calibrator. This is then repeated with the vial only, removing the lead container. The lead will absorb virtually all of the 140 keV gamma rays from the $^{99}Tc^m$, but only 50% of the 740 keV gamma rays from the ^{99}Mo. Comparing the ionisation current readings allows calculation of the level of ^{99}Mo present in the eluate. The maximum permitted level of ^{99}Mo in the sample is one part per 1000.

Radiochemical Purity

This measures the proportion of the total activity present in the stated chemical form. Possible contaminants in $^{99}Tc^m$ labelled radiopharmaceuticals are free pertechnetate, $^{99}Tc^mO_4$, and reduced forms of $^{99}Tc^m$. The purity is measured using thin-layer chromatography.

- A drop of the radiopharmaceutical is applied at the bottom of the chromatogram
- This is placed in a solvent, ensuring that the origin is not immersed
- As the solvent migrates along the chromatogram, different chemical species in the radiopharmaceutical are separated

The chromatogram is then analysed to calculate the percentage of bound, free, and reduced $^{99}Tc^{m}$ in the preparation. For radiopharmaceuticals, radiochemical purity should be >95%.

Chemical Purity

This measures the fraction of the total mass present in the sample, which is in the stated chemical form. The main possible chemical contaminant of $^{99}Tc^{m}$ is Al^{3+} from the alumina column in the generator. Aluminium concentration is tested on the first elution of the generator using a commercially available kit. This contains Al^{3+} indicator papers and a standard Al^{3+} solution of 10 mg/mL. A drop of the standard is placed on the indicator paper next to a drop from the eluate. The intensity of the colour produced by the eluate should be less than that produced by the standard.

Sterility

All substances for patient injection must be tested to ensure sterility. Surplus eluate (after decay) and samples of each radiopharmaceutical (after decay) are sent to bacteriology for testing. Due to the short shelf life of $^{99}Tc^{m}$ radiopharmaceuticals, preparations have to be released prior to the results of sterility testing being known. Testing can only show that the product was sterile at the time of testing, not at the time of use. Testing for pyrogens may also be carried out. Pyrogens are polysaccharides which may be the metabolic products of bacteria, yeasts, and fungi. Demonstrating that a sample achieves the required level of sterility is not a guarantee of apyrogenicity.

Technetium-99m Generator

As has previously been mentioned, $^{99}Tc^{m}$ is obtained from a radionuclide generator containing ^{99}Mo. This decays to $^{99}Tc^{m}$ with a half-life of 2.8 days (67.2 hours) by beta decay, as seen in Fig. 1.27. The optimal working life of a generator is around seven to ten days. Although some activity can be extracted beyond this time, it is unlikely to be sufficient for a full day's activity in a busy nuclear medicine department. Generators are generally referenced by the activity they will produce on a given date, which will typically be tens of gigabecquerels. The generator can be used before this date, but this will reduce the activity available later in its working lifespan. Many departments will get their generators delivered at the weekend or early on a Monday morning to allow optimal production capacity at the beginning of the working week.

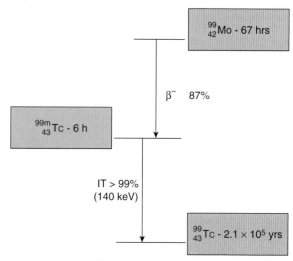

Fig. 1.27 Simplified decay series of molybdenum-99.

The activity of $^{99}Tc^{m}$ available for extraction from the generator increases as more ^{99}Mo nuclei decay. The process of extraction is known as the elution of the generator and involves the washing of a solution of sterile saline over the ceramic column to which the ^{99}Mo is adhered. Fig. 1.28 shows a simple schematic of the components of the generator. Immediately after each elution, the activity of $^{99}Tc^{m}$ remaining in the generator is reduced to zero, as shown in Fig. 1.29. By a happy coincidence, the half-lives of the parent and daughter in the technetium generator mean that the maximum activity of $^{99}Tc^{m}$ is achieved approximately 24 hours after the last elution, which fits in very well with the working day. Over several days, the maximum available activity of $^{99}Tc^{m}$ decreases with the decay of the parent ^{99}Mo.

For this reason, larger departments may get a second delivery of a smaller generator in the middle of the week to maintain the supply level in the second half of the week. The alternative is to front-load the week with the studies requiring higher activity levels, but this reduces flexibility and can be logistically very difficult.

Mechanisms of Radiopharmaceutical Localisation

The vast majority of radiopharmaceuticals in routine use in nuclear medicine are labelled with $^{99}Tc^{m}$ due to its superior imaging characteristics and ready availability. The number of non-technetium radiopharmaceuticals in use has decreased in recent years as manufacturers have developed technetium-labelled replacements to make use of these advantages. However, a number of non-technetium radiopharmaceuticals remain due to their

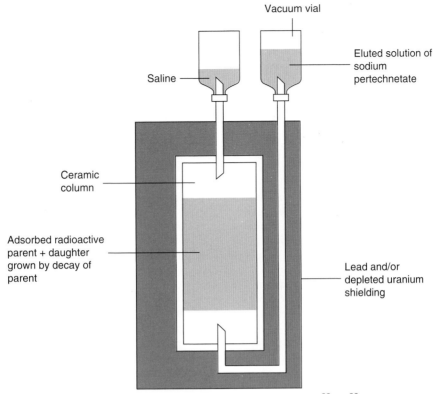

Fig. 1.28 Simplified schematic diagram of the components of a ^{99}Mo/^{99}Tc^m generator.

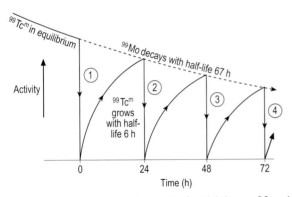

Fig. 1.29 Graph of the activity levels of molybdenum-99 and technetium-99m within a ^{99}Mo/^{99}Tc^m generator, which is being eluted at 24 h intervals.

specific characteristics and methods by which they function physiologically. The biochemical and physiological methods by which radiopharmaceuticals reach their target organs are fundamental to the success of nuclear medicine as an imaging technique, and a number of these will now be described in detail.

Facilitated Diffusion

Physiological factors of the pharmaceutical, such as lipophilicity, favour passive transport through a lipid membrane. The primary example of this in nuclear medicine is the imaging of cerebral blood flow by use of ^{99}Tc^m hexamethylpropyleneamineoxime. This is lipophilic, so it passes through the blood/brain barrier, but once in the brain and subject to a different biochemical environment, it converts to a hydrophilic compound that is essentially 'locked in' and cannot pass back through the membrane.

Active Transport Mechanisms

These are methods of uptake where energy is consumed during the transport process. The energy consumption can allow transport across a concentration gradient. One example is during the uptake of ^{201}Tl by the myocardium. The thallous ions are taken up by the transport mechanism for potassium via the sodium-potassium pump with the energy provided by adenosine triphosphate. This has the advantage that uptake of the radiopharmaceutical by the myocytes directly reflects myocardial blood flow.

However, the poor characteristics of ^{201}Tl (long half-life, low-energy gamma emissions, etc.) result in a high radiation dose to the patient. It has generally been superseded by ^{99}Tc^m labelled isonitrile compounds such as sestamibi and tetrofosmin. Uptake of these does not linearly relate to blood flow, but the imaging and radiation dose advantages greatly outweigh this.

Capillary Trapping

This method relies on the physical trapping of the molecules of the radiopharmaceutical within small blood vessels by nature of their physical size. Intravenous injection of a particulate suspension with particles of diameter >10−15 μm results in the trapping of these particles in the pulmonary capillary bed. The most common example of this is technetium-99m macroaggregated albumin lung perfusion studies, where 1 mg of human albumin in the form of microspheres 60−90 μm in diameter blocks a maximum of 0.3% of available pulmonary vessels in a normal subject. This allows sufficient activity to obtain diagnostic images in a short time frame whilst posing no significant risk to most patients.

Receptor Binding

The utilisation of receptor sites on molecules offers the possibility for highly specific radiotracers. For example, the neuropeptide somatostatin can be radiolabelled with ^{111}In pentetreotide and used to image tumours with somatostatin receptors, such as carcinoids, pancreatic endocrine tumours, neuroblastomas, and paragangliomas. This has been replaced to some extent by ^{99}Tc^m labelled Tektrotyd, which binds to a very similar subset of receptor sites and has the advantages of being technetium labelled.

Another common example is imaging the transport of dopamine through the brain using ^{123}I-FPCIT, known as DaTscan. This demonstrates the dopamine transporter sites within the synapse and is very useful for distinguishing between idiopathic Parkinson's disease and associated syndromes such as essential tremor.

Compartmental Localisation and Leakage

Compartmental localisation refers to the introduction of the radiopharmaceutical into a well-defined anatomic compartment, such as ^{81}Kr^m gas inhalation into the lung.

Compartmental leakage is used to identify an abnormal opening in an otherwise closed compartment, such as the use of ^{99}Tc^m labelled red blood cells to detect gastrointestinal bleeding.

Physiochemical Adsorption

The most common example of this method is the use of diphosphonate compounds, where localisation occurs primarily by adsorption into the mineral structure of the bone. The diphosphonate concentrations are significantly higher in amorphous calcium than in mature hydroxyapatite crystalline structures, which helps to explain their concentration in areas of increased osteogenic activity. This produces an image containing 'hotspots' that are more easily detected by the human visual system than 'cold spots' produced by purely lytic processes.

Methylene diphosphonate and hydroxyl diphosphonate are the most widely available pharmaceuticals for bone imaging and perform similarly, although with slightly different clearance rates from soft tissue.

Phagocytosis

Uptake by phagocytosis occurs when particles of 25Å to 10 mm diameter are engulfed by phagocytic cells such as the Kupffer cells of the liver or the macrophages of the spleen and bone marrow. This is brought about by the recognition of the particle by receptors on the cell surface. One example is the use of ^{99}Tc^m tin and sulphur colloids for liver scanning.

Metabolic Incorporation

As mentioned earlier, radionuclides of specific elements follow identical metabolic pathways to non-radioactive nuclides. Therefore, ^{123}I can be used for thyroid imaging as much of the iodine taken up into the body is concentrated in the thyroid.

The positron emitter fluorine-18 in the chemical form of fluorodeoxyglucose (FDG) is a glucose analogue, and its uptake into cells correlates with their glucose metabolism. This is extremely important for oncology imaging as cancer cells have elevated levels of glucose metabolism.

Chemotaxis

Chemotaxis describes the movement of a cell, such as a leukocyte, in response to a chemical stimulus. Therefore, ^{99}Tc^m labelled leucocytes (white cells) respond to products formed in immunologic reactions by migrating and accumulating at the site of the reaction as part of an overall inflammatory response. This allows imaging of infective and inflammatory processes such as graft infection, prosthetic joint infection, or inflammatory bowel diseases.

Sequestration

The main use of this method is where autologous platelet cells labelled with ^{111}In are injected, and the site of removal (i.e. sequestration) is evaluated. In patients with idiopathic thrombocytopaenia (ITP), the ratio between splenic and liver sequestration at 5 days determines whether splenectomy is a valid treatment option.

FURTHER READING

Aufbau principle, Double slit experiment, Jablonski diagram, Triplet state.

REFERENCES

1. Medicines and Healthcare Products Regulatory Agency and Department of Health and Social Care. *Good Manufacturing Practice and Good Distribution Practice*; 2020 [Online]. Available at: https://www.gov.uk/guidance/good-manufacturing-practice-and-good-distribution-practice#overview (Accessed: 05 May 2022).
2. UK Statutory Instruments. *The Human Medicines Regulations*; 2012 [Online]. Available at: https://www.legislation.gov.uk/uksi/2012/1916/contents/made (Accessed: 05 May 2022).
3. UK Statutory Instruments. *The Ionising Radiations Regulations*; 2017 [Online]. Available at: https://www.legislation.gov.uk/uksi/2017/1075/contents/made (Accessed: 05 May 2022).

2

Radiation Hazards and Protection

CHAPTER CONTENTS

INTERACTIONS OF IONISING RADIATION WITH TISSUE

Ionising radiation is particularly hazardous to tissue as the interactions occur on the atomic scale. The ionisation of a single atom generates approximately 35 eV of energy, which is significantly greater than the energy of a covalent bond in a strand of DNA, which is around 4 eV, or the energy of a hydrogen bond holding together strands of DNA, which is approximately 0.4 eV. The secondary electrons generated by the ionisation of an atom will cause further ionisations. These clusters of ionisation, often known as ionisation events, can cause significant damage on the atomic scale. These events are common when alpha particles interact with tissue, are less common when beta particles interact, and are rare when gamma or X-rays interact with tissue.

Ionising radiation causes damage to the biological molecules of tissue via two mechanisms:

- Breaking molecular bonds directly via the energy released from ionisation events
- Ionising water molecules within the tissue to produce H^+ ions and $OH^•$ free radicals, which then damage biological molecules

Given that water is the predominant constituent of soft tissue, it can be estimated that the $OH^•$ free radicals are responsible for around two-thirds of the damage caused to tissue by gamma or X-rays.

The most serious damage to biological cells caused by ionising radiation is DNA damage. Damage to DNA is involved in acute injury after high-dose exposures and is associated with a greater risk of future cancers after low-dose exposures. Adjacent breaks in both strands of a DNA molecule are particularly important in terms of biological damage. However, biological damage is not exclusive to DNA and can also involve cell membranes.

Radiation exposure, or dose, is characterised by the absorbed dose which describes the amount of energy deposited in a unit mass of tissue and is measured in grays (Gy).

$$1 \text{ gray} = 1 \text{ joule per kg}$$

1 Gy is a high dose of radiation generally only encountered in radiotherapy for destruction of malignant tissues. In medical imaging applications, the doses encountered are generally of the order of μGy or mGy.

Cell survival curves are a means of assessing the damage caused by radiation exposure. The proportion of a cell population surviving after radiation exposure is compared to an identical, non-irradiated control population and plotted against the radiation dose. As seen in Fig. 2.1, these can be plotted for different types of radiation with the cell death efficiency reflecting the amount of ionisation caused by each type of radiation.

This can be quantified by use of linear energy transfer (LET), which is dependent on the type of radiation and its energy. This describes the density of ionisation along the track of the radiation.

Low-LET radiation: 0.2—10 keV/mm deposited energy X-rays, gamma rays, beta particles

High-LET radiation: 10—100 keV/mm alpha particles, neutrons

Alpha particles and neutrons produce dense ionisation and are likely to damage both strands of a DNA molecule, which cannot be repaired. The less ionising X-rays are likely only to damage a single strand, which is more readily repaired by the body's repair mechanisms.

Radiation weighting factors (w_R) can be defined which indicate the effectiveness of radiation in causing damage to biological tissue (see Table 2.1). As shown later, these can be used to calculate the equivalent dose of radiation to which a subject has been exposed.

These weighting factors can be used to define the effectiveness of radiation exposures in damaging biological tissue. They are used to adjust the absorbed dose in Gy into an equivalent dose H_T which is measured in sieverts (Sv).

$$H_T = \sum w_R D_R$$

As in most medical uses of radiation, we will be using radiations with a w_R of 1; therefore, the equivalent dose in Sv is of the same magnitude as the absorbed dose in Gy.

The route of exposure must also be considered in hazard assessment. As alpha particles deposit their energy very rapidly, they do not penetrate very far through skin and do not present a great hazard from external exposure. Conversely, if they are ingested or inhaled into the body, they can cause considerable damage to internal tissues, such as the lining of the lungs. Therefore, the hazard posed by different radiation types must be differentiated based on the route of exposure. This is described in Table 2.2.

Neutrons are not used medically but are produced by particle accelerators such as linear accelerators and cyclotrons, which may be present in the hospital environment. Neutrons interact with the protons of hydrogen atoms within the tissue and are therefore more penetrating than alpha particles. Organic polymers with high densities of hydrogen atoms, such as polythene, can be used as shielding material around these.

The rate at which a radiation exposure occurs, or dose rate, must also be considered when determining the damage that a specific radiation dose can cause.

At low dose rates, the tissue repair mechanisms can repair DNA damage prior to the next exposure, but the cumulative damage defeats these mechanisms at higher dose rates and cell death is more likely to occur. Therefore, more cells are killed per unit dose at high dose rates, as seen in Fig. 2.2.

The distribution of a high dose into numerous smaller fractions delivered with fixed time intervals between them, known as fractionation, also affects the damage caused to tissue, as seen in Fig. 2.3.

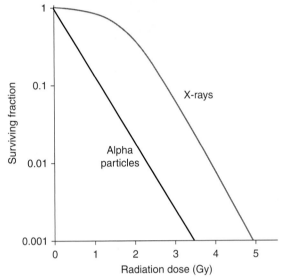

Fig. 2.1 Variation in cell survival after exposure to doses of alpha particles and X-rays.

TABLE 2.1 Radiation Weighting Factors for Different Types of Radiation	
Type of Radiation	Radiation Weighting Factor w_R
X-rays and gamma rays	1
Beta particles and positrons	1
Alpha particles	20
Neutrons	5–20, dependent on energy

TABLE 2.2 Effectiveness of Radiation at Causing Biological Damage Depending on the Route of Exposure			
Route of Exposure	*Most Effective*		*Least Effective*
Internal	Alpha particles	Beta particles	X-rays and gamma rays
External	X-rays and gamma rays	Beta particles	Alpha particles

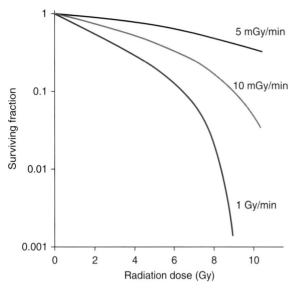

Fig. 2.2 Difference in cell survival depending on dose rate.

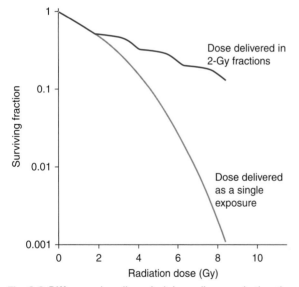

Fig. 2.3 Difference in cell survival depending on whether the dose is administered as a single acute dose or as 2-Gy fractions separated by 18 hours each time.

Separating exposures by intervals of greater than 12 hours allows for tissue repair to occur between them. As healthy tissues generally have more effective repair mechanisms than tumours, this can be utilised in radiotherapy to maximise tumour killing while sparing damage to surrounding healthy tissues.

TABLE 2.3	Radiosensitivities of Different Tissue Types	
High	**Medium**	**Low**
Bone marrow	Skin	Muscle
Gastrointestinal system	Liver	Bones
Breast tissue	Lungs	Nervous system
Gonads	Kidneys	Blood vessels

The rate of division of various cell types generally determines their sensitivity to a specific dose of radiation. The faster cell types are dividing, the greater their radiosensitivity, meaning that the sensitivity of different tissue types is a function of the component cell types within the tissue. Table 2.3 shows the distribution of radiosensitivities for a variety of tissue types.

As can be seen, organs with higher cell proliferation are most sensitive, whilst those with the most static cell populations are the least sensitive.

From a radiation protection perspective, the cells' ability to repair is not the only factor to be considered. There are also biological mechanisms to stop damaged cells from replicating which must be considered. There are two methods by which cells with damage to both DNA strands may be controlled:
- The cell may be prevented from dividing for a period to allow repair to be attempted
- The cell may undergo programmed cell death or apoptosis

Apoptosis is generally used to control cells which are no longer required but can also be used to remove damaged cells.

Mechanisms of cell repair are not foolproof, and errors in repair of DNA strands may be missed by the control methods described above, allowing damaged cells to propagate. This may be of greater long-term risk than acute cell death, as these damaged cells may develop into cancers in the longer term. This risk may be related to changes in specific genes which control cell growth, differentiation, and proliferation, causing errors in gene expression and cell regulation. There is a finite probability of these events occurring even at very low doses of radiation exposure.

Effects of Radiation Exposure

The average person in the UK is exposed to an effective dose of 2.7 mSv per year from background radiation.

Around 2.3 mSv of this is from natural sources in the environment and the remainder is from medical exposures.

The natural component of background radiation comes from four main sources, which are:

Cosmic — Radiation from the Sun and space which has penetrated the Earth's protective magnetic field. Cosmic radiation increases with altitude, and so the highest exposures for most will come during long-haul flights (i.e., a transatlantic flight produces an exposure of ~0.04 mSv).

Terrestrial — Radiation from rocks and soil and their incorporation into building materials. The bulk of the exposure is from radioactive actinium, thorium, and uranium and their decay products. This can vary widely between regions depending upon local geology.

Radon — Radioactive gas which is part of the decay of uranium-238. It is an alpha-particle emitter and some of its daughter products are also alpha-particle emitters. It therefore accounts for around 50% of an average person's annual background exposure in the UK. This also varies widely with location and is highest in regions with a large proportion of granite in the local geology such as Cornwall and Royal Deeside.

Food — A variety of plants contain naturally occurring radionuclides (as does the human body), such as potassium-40 in bananas and polonium-210 in tobacco leaves. There has also been incorporation of radionuclides such as iodine-131 and caesium-137 into foodstuffs from environmental atomic bomb tests in the 1950s and 1960s.

Much of the data available on the effects of ionising radiation on the human body comes from animal studies and from studies of the survivors of nuclear incidents, such as the bombings of Hiroshima and Nagasaki and the reactor meltdown at Chernobyl. The effects can be split into two main categories:

Deterministic effects — Also known as tissue effects which occur rapidly (i.e., hours to weeks) after exposure to high doses of radiation. These generally occur above a threshold dose which depends on the tissue type.

Stochastic effects — These occur many years after exposure, if at all. The probability of occurrence is small but increases with the dose received.

Deterministic Effects

Table 2.4 shows the threshold doses for deterministic effects in a variety of tissues.

Acute whole-body exposures to high doses, such as those experienced by the firefighters at Chernobyl, can cause radiation sickness. The symptoms of this include vomiting, diarrhoea, reduced blood count, and haemorrhage, and can lead to death.

Table 2.5 shows the whole-body doses associated with radiation sickness. In the absence of medical treatment, the lowest dose likely to cause death is around 3–5 Sv. However, treatments such as bone marrow transplants can alleviate these risks to some extent.

In the skin, the basal epidermis is the most radiosensitive and the first direct effect is erythema, which occurs at doses of around 2–5 Gy. These are levels which can be

TABLE 2.5 Whole-Body Doses and Their Mean Time to Death by Acute Radiation Sickness

Whole-Body Absorbed Dose (Gy)	Tissue Involved	Time from Exposure to Death (days)
1–6	Bone marrow	30–60
5–15	Gastrointestinal tract	10–20
>15	Central nervous system	1–5

TABLE 2.4 Threshold Doses for Tissue Effects in Various Tissue Types

Tissue	Effect	Absorbed Dose (Gy)	Development Time
Skin	Initial erythema	2	2–24 h
	Erythema	3–6	1–4 weeks
	Temporary hair loss	3–4	2–3 weeks
Lens of eye	Cataract	3–5	Several years
Bone marrow	Depression of blood cell production	0.5	3–7 days
Gonads	Temporary male sterility	0.15	3–9 weeks
	Permanent sterility	3.5–6	3 weeks

encountered in the medical environment in areas such as radiotherapy and fluoroscopic procedures in interventional radiology and cardiac catheterisation.

The lens of the eye is also sensitive to radiation exposures, and coagulation of proteins within the lens can occur at doses over 2 Gy. This causes opacities within the lens, which are cumulative, and over time can lead to vision impairment due to cataracts.

Stochastic Effects

These are random effects which obey the laws of probability. The impact of the effect does not increase with increasing dose but the likelihood of it occurring does increase with dose. There are two types of stochastic effects:

- Induction of cancer in a subject exposed to radiation
- Production of genetic abnormalities in the offspring of the subject or subsequent generations (heritable effects)

Many of the epidemiological studies carried out to examine stochastic effects have used data from the atomic bomb survivors of Hiroshima and Nagasaki and from accidents such as Chernobyl. These populations were exposed to high doses, but their study has several limitations which have led to uncertainty and disagreement about the exact effects of radiation, as will be discussed. To minimise the risk of stochastic effects, data from these studies has been used to develop dose limits, as will be discussed later.

The heritable effects of exposures have been studied using animal models, but data is now available from the offspring of those exposed in Japan and at Chernobyl, which indicates that there are no discernible effects at the level of statistical significance obtainable from the population sizes available. However, these have shown that there are direct effects other than cancer induction, with some evidence of increased risk of cardiovascular and cerebrovascular disease.

The data from the atomic bomb survivors is important as it demonstrates the effects of whole-body irradiation over a range of doses and ages at exposure. These demonstrate that the risk of cancer induction increases with dose and in an almost linear fashion for solid tumours. The difficulty arising from this is that the statistically significant increase in risk only begins above doses of 100−200 mSv, which are well above those from most medical exposures. The risk increases in a quadratic fashion for the induction of leukaemia, but again, there is a threshold dose of 100−200 mSv.

The model recommended by the International Commission on Radiological Protection (ICRP) for calculation of risk is the linear−no threshold (LNT) model,[1] as seen in Fig. 2.4. This is simple to apply but implies that there is no

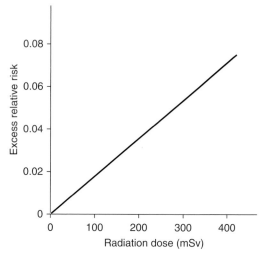

Fig. 2.4 Example of risk associated with exposure calculated using the linear non-threshold model.

safe dose of radiation, which contradicts the evidence of a threshold dose from the atomic bomb data as discussed above.

However, there is considerable disagreement about the applicability of the LNT model as most of the exposures involved in the data were considerably above those experienced in most medical applications, often by orders of magnitude. Different models for extrapolating to low-dose exposures have been proposed using different mathematical models but none has been widely accepted as being better than the prevailing LNT model. It is generally very difficult to assess the risks from low-level radiation exposures as the effects are so small that massive population numbers are required, and groups of exposed and unexposed subjects have to be matched. None of the groups which have been assessed, such as nuclear workers, are large enough to avoid the effects of confounding variables, such as smoking history, among others.

It is also the case that different ethnic and regional populations have markedly different natural incidences of various cancers. This also leads to controversy around the validity of using modelling based on a particular population in a wider group. It also leads to the concepts of absolute and relative risk, defined as follows:

Absolute risk − assumes a constant excess risk after a particular latent period

Relative risk − risk relative to the natural incidence of the cancer in the population, considering age and other effects

The latent period and the differences in risk of cancer induction in different tissues were some of the most important results to come from studies of atomic bomb survivors. The latent period was short, at around 5–15 years for leukaemia but was generally much greater than 10 years for solid tumours.

The age at exposure was also an important factor, and it was found that the risk was highest in children under 10 years at the time of exposure due to the higher cell division rate associated with growth and longer remaining lifetime. The risk then drops with increasing age until it effectively plateaus between the ages of 30 and 60, and then drops again in those over 60 due to the limited time remaining for cancers to develop. There are particular risks with foetal exposure, especially in the first two trimesters. Exposure at these stages can cause mental retardation with resultant low IQ and there is also an increased risk of the development of childhood cancers.

Effective Dose

Most exposures to radiation, especially in medical applications, will not be distributed uniformly throughout the body. As discussed earlier, different tissues have varying sensitivities to radiation exposure, and a method of calculating a relative risk from any exposure was developed by the ICRP, whereby tissues are assigned different weighting factors. These are based on the best available evidence and are reviewed regularly. The weighting factors sum to 1 so that they represent a weighted sum of doses to radiosensitive organs.

The effective dose gives an indication of risk for any exposure based on a uniform whole-body dose that would produce a similar risk to the actual dose distribution to which the individual was subjected. The calculation of risk to health includes the probability of inducing a fatal cancer, the weighted probability of inducing a non-fatal cancer, the relative length of any reduction in lifespan, and the probability of severe hereditary disease. It is calculated as:

$$Effective\ dose = \sum(H_T \times w_T)$$

where H_T is the equivalent dose to each tissue and w_T is the tissue weighting factor for that tissue.

It should be highlighted that effective dose can only be computed. It cannot be measured directly. To allow computation, mathematical modelling techniques are used to derive coefficients which enable organ doses to be calculated using quantities which can be measured in medical exposures, such as the dose-area product (DAP) for X-ray examinations. Due to uncertainties in the modelling, the relative accuracy for any individual patient exposure is around ±50%.

TABLE 2.6 Suggested Terms for the Risks Likely at a Range of Doses

Effective Dose (mSv)	Risk
<0.1	Negligible
0.1–1	Minimal
1–10	Very low
10–100	Low

The concept of effective dose is based on the LNT model which gives a 5% excess risk of developing a cancer per sievert of dose. The uncertainties in this and the modelling result in a system where risk can only be described within orders of magnitude (i.e., 1 in 10,000 or 1 in 1,000).

For this reason, it is generally the case that the terms shown in Table 2.6 are used to describe the risk associated with particular dose ranges.

The general population often find it difficult to comprehend the concepts of relative risk and it is therefore often helpful to equate these to risks with which they will be more familiar in everyday life. These can include risks from flying or driving certain distances or those from lifestyle choices such as smoking.

RADIATION PROTECTION

Fundamental Principles

The assimilation of scientific knowledge and research around exposure to ionising radiation and the development of this into recommendations for radiation protection is carried out by several bodies, but the most influential is the ICRP. This was founded in 1928 and works with groups from the UN, World Health Organisation (WHO), and the International Atomic Energy Agency (IAEA) to assimilate evidence from expert advisory groups and develop consensus guidance. This is necessary as there is little direct evidence of harm at low-level exposures. The guidance developed is generally pragmatic and conservative in nature and expressed in general rather than specific form to allow interpretation and implementation into local legislation.

There are three main tenets to radiation protection guidance:
- All practices involving ionising radiation should be justified
- All practices involving ionising radiation should be optimised

- Notwithstanding these, there are limits to the exposure of an individual which cannot be exceeded

Justification

This is defined in ICRP Report 60[2] as:

> *No practice involving exposures to radiation should be adopted unless it produces sufficient benefit to the exposed individuals or to society to offset the radiation detriment it causes.*

The process of justification of generic procedures in the UK is undertaken by the Royal College of Radiologists (RCR) in their guidelines. These use a traffic light system to recommend the preferred and acceptable imaging techniques for given patient conditions. They also indicate which techniques are not appropriate and discuss the reasoning behind the recommendations. These guidelines are now available on-line at the iRefer website (https://www.irefer.org.uk/).

The justification of individual patient exposures falls under the Ionising Radiation (Medical Exposure) Regulations (IR(ME)R) 2017[3] and will be described in detail later in this chapter.

Optimisation

The principle aim of optimisation is to maximise the benefit gained from the radiation exposure whilst minimising the harm that arises from it. In imaging, this must also take account of the exposure required to obtain adequate image quality. This can be a complicated process and the advice of specialist radiation protection professionals may be required.

The general principle of optimisation can be expressed in broad terms as ensuring that any exposure is 'as low as reasonably achievable', which is known as the ALARA principle. This is also sometimes defined as 'as low as reasonably practicable', or ALARP.

Limits

Dose limits are set by regulatory bodies to ensure that individuals are protected. Thus, any practice which has been justified and optimised still cannot exceed the dose limit set.

It should be highlighted that dose limits do not apply to patients undergoing medical exposures, or to those looking after them, who are known in the legislation as 'carers and comforters'. Exposures to patients are minimised through diagnostic reference levels (DRLs), as will be described later. The protection of carers and comforters is achieved by setting constraints, which are restrictions on the range of options which can be considered for the process of dose optimisation. In general terms, these are usually a fraction of the dose limit applicable.

There are three principles which should always be applied in practical radiation protection:
- Time — The longer the exposure to a source, the higher the dose received. Therefore, exposure time should always be minimised.
- Distance — The radiation dose decreases with distance away from the source, according to the inverse square law (i.e., if you double the distance, the dose drops to one-quarter).
- Shielding — This is material placed around the source to attenuate the radiation and reduce the exposure to those nearby. High-density materials such as lead, tungsten, and concrete (potentially doped with boron) are ideal for this purpose.

Principles of Dosimetry

Thus far, we have talked about exposure without clearly defining it. Ionising radiation passing through any material generates secondary electrons. As these slow down and stop, they deposit energy as charge in the material. Exposure, X, is defined in air as the charge deposited in a unit mass when all the electrons have stopped. Therefore,

$$X = dQ/dm$$

This is measured in coulombs per kilogram (Ckg^{-1}), but this is not a particularly useful unit for practical radiation protection.

The parameter which is more useful is that of the kinetic energy of the charged particles released by the passage of the ionising radiation through a unit mass of material. This kinetic energy released per unit mass (KERMa) is defined as:

$$Kerma = dE/dm$$

and is measured in joules per kilogram (Jkg^{-1}), which as we have seen earlier has units of Gy. At diagnostic energies, of up to around 140 keV, air kerma is used to define the output of X-ray sets, typically expressed in mGy/mAs at a distance of one metre.

The fundamental quantity of dosimetry in practical radiation protection is the **absorbed dose** to tissue, or D_T. This also describes the energy deposited by the charged particles liberated by the radiation as it passes through a unit mass of material and therefore, as we saw earlier, also has units of Gy. This is generally averaged over the organ or tissue which is being considered. Both kerma and absorbed dose are measurable quantities.

The **equivalent dose** is a calculated parameter, measured in Sv, produced by multiplying the measured absorbed dose by a weighting factor for the relative biological effectiveness of the radiation, as we saw earlier.

We use another calculated parameter to estimate the stochastic risk from any exposure: the **effective dose.** As we have seen earlier, this is the sum of the equivalent dose to each tissue multiplied by a tissue weighting factor dependent upon its radiosensitivity. It represents the uniform whole-body dose which produces the same radiation risk as the non-uniform absorbed dose and is also measured in Sv.

The dose limits set by legislation are defined using effective dose for whole-body exposures and equivalent dose for the limits to particular organs, such as the fingers or the lens of the eye.

LEGISLATION

Although the UK is no longer part of the EU, the UK legislation regarding radiation protection remains closely aligned. There are two main pieces of legislation dealing with the protection of staff and the public, and the patients, respectively. These will be dealt with in turn.

Ionising Radiation Regulations (IRR) 2017[4]

These describe the legislation to be followed to minimise exposures to the public and employees and sit under the Health and Safety at Work Act 1974. The enforcement body for these is the Health and Safety Executive (HSE). These apply to all work with ionising radiation, not just medical applications. They are designed to ensure that all exposures are ALARP and below the limits defined in the regulations.

They are supported by an Approved Code of Practice[5] (ACOP) which is published by the HSE. If you follow the ACOP, then you are deemed to be compliant with the regulations. However, if you do not follow the ACOP, you will be required to demonstrate how you are compliant with the regulations in other ways. There are other forms of guidance, such as the Medical and Dental Guidance Notes[6] (MDGN), which are published by the Institute of Physics and Engineering in Medicine (IPEM). However, these are subtly different from the ACOP in that they describe good practice, but following them does not legally deem that you are compliant with the regulations in the way that following the ACOP does.

There are 43 regulations set out in 7 sections within the document. The employer is the main duty holder and is responsible for ensuring compliance, but there are also duties on employees as well which may be enforceable by law. The employer must appoint a Radiation Protection Adviser (RPA) to advise them on how to comply with the regulations. The RPA must be appointed in writing and must hold a certificate of competence from the approved body. That is RPA 2000 in the UK, and they are responsible for setting out the curriculum which must be followed and examining the submitted portfolios by those wishing to obtain RPA certification.

In each area designated for the use of ionising radiation, there must also be a suitably qualified Radiation Protection Supervisor (RPS) appointed and a set of local rules drawn up which set out the local procedures to ensure compliance with the regulations. The RPS is responsible for ensuring that the local rules are followed in practical terms within their area of responsibility.

It is good practice for the employer to have a radiation safety policy which is available to all staff and a radiation safety committee which meets regularly to review all issues related to compliance with the regulations. The membership of this should contain the senior manager with delegated responsibility for compliance with all relevant radiation protection legislation, who will be advised by the RPA. Membership will also contain RPSs from relevant areas of the organisation and responsible persons from relevant sectors, such as health and safety.

Other Duties

Training — It is a duty of the employer to ensure that all staff who may be exposed to ionising radiation are suitably trained for working with it. The RPA will advise to ensure that the training is suited to the needs of each individual and relevant to their area of work.

Pregnancy — It is a duty of the employer to ensure that all pregnant staff are fully aware of the risks arising from ionising radiation to their foetus or nursing infant if they are breastfeeding. It is the duty of the pregnant employee to notify their employer in writing as soon as they have confirmed their pregnancy or if they are breastfeeding when they return to work.

Equipment — It is a duty of equipment manufacturers which use ionising radiation to ensure that they are designed and constructed in a way that minimises potential exposure to staff and other persons as far as is practicable. It is a duty of the installers of these pieces of equipment to ensure that all warning lights and safety features are working as designed after installation. This is done by carrying out a critical examination which may be done in conjunction with, or supervised by, the RPA. The installer is also responsible for passing on all relevant information for the safe use, testing, and maintenance of the equipment.

Employees — It is a duty of the employee to wear any dosimeter provided to them by the employer and to wear appropriately any personal protective equipment (PPE) provided. They must also report any faults with PPE or dosimeters and return them to their correct location after use. They must also report any suspected radiation incidents to the employer and behave in an appropriate manner when working with ionising radiation to reduce the risks to themselves and others.

Radiation Risk Assessments (RRAs) are a fundamental part of the processes which must be undertaken to ensure compliance with IRR. An RRA must be carried out before any new activity involving ionising radiation is carried out. The RRA should identify the potential hazards, recommend measures to restrict exposures and, if necessary, state whether restrictions to access are required.

To assist in carrying out RRAs, there are 5 basic steps which should be considered:

- Identify the potential hazards
- Identify those who may be at risk of being harmed
- Evaluate the risks and decide on the precautions required
- Record these in a controlled document and implement the recommendations
- Review the risk assessment and precautions after a reasonable period and update the RRA if required

The employer is responsible for restricting the exposure to staff and the public, consistent with the principle of ALARA. To achieve this, a hierarchy of control is required by the regulations:

- Firstly, doses should be restricted using engineering controls and design features and through safety features and warning devices.
- After applying these, systems of work should be applied to support these.
- When it is practicable, the employer should also provide PPE to further reduce exposure.

The employer must also use dose constraints, take special precautions for pregnant and breastfeeding staff, and set dose investigation levels.

The dose investigation levels will generally be determined with the input of the RPA and should be appropriate to the work of the staff in the area. They are set out in the local rules for the area and will initiate a review of working conditions when they are exceeded. Legally, an investigation must be carried out the first time a staff member receives a dose of greater than 15 mSv in a year. However, this will be set considerably below this value in most healthcare settings.

After a staff member has informed their employer that they are pregnant, the employer must ensure that the equivalent dose to the foetus is less than 1 mSv for the remainder of the duration of the pregnancy. An RRA, either existing or newly carried out, should be used to determine any restrictions or changes to working practice that are required to achieve this. If the staff member works with unsealed radioactive sources, such as radiopharmaceuticals in a nuclear medicine department, then risks due to breastfeeding must also be considered. The employer is again only responsible once informed by the staff member that they are breastfeeding, but it is best practice for the employer to consider this to be the case for 6 months after the return to work regardless. Staff should always be encouraged to notify the employer in writing, as this formally records the responsibility. Again, an RRA should be used to determine any actions required. The breastfeeding infant is subject to the same dose limits as a member of the public and the employer may choose to apply a dose constraint at a fraction of this limit.

Dose Limits

There are three main categories of people who must be considered for the setting of dose limits:

Employees over 18 years of age: the limit on whole-body effective dose is 20 mSv per year

The equivalent dose limit to the lens of the eye is 20 mSv per year, or in certain circumstances can be 100 Sv over a 5-year period subject to a maximum of 50 mSv in any calendar year

The equivalent dose limits for the skin and extremities are 500 mSv per year

Trainees under 18: the limit on whole-body effective dose is 6 mSv per year

The equivalent dose limit to the lens of the eye is 15 mSv per year

The equivalent dose limits for the skin and extremities are 150 mSv per year

Other persons: the limit on whole-body effective dose is 1 mSv per year

The equivalent dose limit to the lens of the eye is 15 mSv per year

The equivalent dose limits for the skin and extremities are 50 mSv per year

This emphasises that it is important to ensure that all persons are categorised appropriately to ensure they are subject to the correct limits. This then leads on to the final category into which staff may be assigned.

If staff are likely to receive an effective dose greater than 6 mSv in a year, or an equivalent dose greater than 15 mSv to the lens of the eye, or greater than 150 mSv per year to the skin or extremities, then the employer must designate them as a classified person.

Classified persons (or workers) must:

- Undergo a medical examination before they are classified and then annually thereafter
- Be over 18 years of age
- Have their dose records kept for a minimum of 30 years by an approved dosimetry service

In the healthcare setting, classified persons are relatively uncommon but may be found amongst interventional radiologists using fluoroscopy techniques and radiopharmacy staff working with radionuclide generators.

Area Designation

Categorisation and designation also applies to the physical environment and controlled and supervised areas may be designated by the employer based on the findings of an RRA. These ensure that exposure restrictions are effective by controlling access to these areas and setting conditions on those entering and working within those areas. Some of the considerations of the RRA will include:

- The type of radiation used within the area
- The external dose rates found in the area
- Likely times of exposure within the area
- Containment and controls within the area, such as shielding or fume cupboards
- The probability of radioactive contamination being generated and the risk of this being spread throughout the area
- The requirement to wear PPE within the area
  An area must be designated as a controlled area if:
- Anyone working in the area is likely to receive an effective dose greater than 6 mSv per year or an equivalent dose greater than 15 mSv per year to the lens of the eye or greater than 150 mSv per year to the skin or extremities
- Any person entering or working in the area is required to follow special procedures to mitigate against significant exposure to ionising radiation or reduce the likelihood or severity of radiation accidents
- The dose rate in the area exceeds 7.5 µSv per hour averaged over the working day
- The dose rate exceeds 7.5 µSv per hour averaged over 1 minute and staff with no radiation protection training are likely to enter the area (this does not apply if the source of the radiation is a patient [i.e., nuclear medicine])
- There is a significant risk of radioactive contamination being present and being transported out with the working area
  An area must be designated as a supervised area if:
- Anyone working in the area is likely to receive an effective dose greater than 1 mSv per year or an equivalent dose greater than 5 mSv per year to the lens of the eye or greater than 50 mSv per year to the skin extremities.

Areas which are under consideration for designation as controlled areas and are being assessed as such may also be designated as supervised areas.

Both controlled and supervised areas must have warning signs where practicable and these should state the nature of the hazard and a contact, often the RPS, for advice. Controlled areas must also have local rules to set out the guidance for work in the areas and should also contain contingency plans to be carried out in the event of accidental exposures. Supervised areas are not required to have local rules but, in the healthcare setting, it is generally considered best practice to have these as well. Both categories of designated areas must also be monitored, using appropriate and well-maintained radiation detection equipment, to ensure that ambient radiation levels are appropriate, that controls are still working, and to detect any leaks or contamination.

The Ionising Radiation (Medical Exposure) Regulations 2017

This is the fundamental legislation for protecting the patient and is based on the principles of justification and optimisation as described earlier. They supersede the original IR(ME)R legislation from 2000 and the older POPUMET rules. However, it does not cover just medical exposures to patients. The full range of indications to which they apply is:

- Diagnostic and therapeutic medical exposures
- Health screening exposures
- Medical research exposures
- Exposures of carers and comforters
- Exposures of asymptomatic persons
- Non-medical exposures carried out using medical radiological equipment

They do not apply uniformly throughout the UK, as Northern Ireland follows the *Ionising Radiation (Medical Exposure) Regulations (Northern Ireland) 2018*,[7] which are enforced by the Regulation and Quality Improvement Authority. In the remaining jurisdictions, the enforcement bodies are as follows:

- England — Care Quality Commission (CQC)
- Scotland — Healthcare Improvement Scotland (HIS)
- Wales — Healthcare Inspectorate Wales (HIW)

There are guidance documents[8] published by the Department of Health and Social Care (DHSC) to guide interpretation, but these do not carry the legal weight of the ACOP under IRR and are guidance only. Further guidance can be found in the MDGN and in publications from other professional bodies.

There are 5 defined roles under IR(ME)R, which are:

- Employer
- Referrer
- Practitioner
- Operator
- Medical physics expert (MPE)

These will now be described in turn.

Employer

The employer is responsible for the implementation of IR(ME)R and for the selection and entitlement of staff to fulfil the defined roles. They must also provide staff with appropriate training, provide written protocols and procedures, and keep an inventory of all equipment associated with medical radiological exposures. The employer is also required to respond in the appropriate manner when an incident has occurred or has the potential to occur.

Referrer

The referrer must be a registered healthcare professional who has been entitled to refer patients for medical exposures. Although most referrers are doctors, they can be from any registered group, such as nurses, clinical scientists, or allied health professionals such as physiotherapists. They must provide enough clinical information on the referral to allow the practitioner to make a reasoned judgement as to the benefit of the procedure.

Practitioner

The practitioner should have had sufficient training and experience to have a detailed knowledge of the benefits and potential harm of all procedures under their scope of practice. A practitioner is required to justify all medical exposures, and an operator should not carry out any exposure until they have adequately confirmed this.

Operator

The operator is responsible for the optimisation of the exposures. This can be by direct involvement with the exposure, such as checking it is the correct patient and selecting the appropriate imaging parameters, or by indirect involvement, such as quality checking the equipment regularly to ensure it is safe for clinical use. They can also authorise exposures if they are following written guidance from a practitioner and they have been appropriately entitled.

MPE

The title of MPE has existed for many years, but IR(ME)R 2017 clarified the role and the requirement for recognition was formalised. It requires the employer to appoint suitably qualified MPEs for all areas involving medical exposures, including nuclear medicine. The level of involvement is determined by the level of hazard and risk from the procedure and the benefit expected from the involvement of the MPE. The legislation also states that the scope of practice of each MPE should be defined in their employer's procedures. This also set out the requirement for all MPEs to be formally certificated through a scheme administered by RPA 2000. In the healthcare setting, MPEs are generally Health and Care Professions Council (HCPC)-registered physicists with the protected title of Clinical Scientist.

Procedures

The employer's written procedures should be maintained under a robust document control system and be authorised by a suitably trained and appropriately entitled person. Some of the more significant procedures include:

Identification of patients — This should detail how the operator should identify the patient, ideally using 3 forms of identification such as name, address, and date of birth. The patient should be prompted to provide these rather than responding to a statement of these. The procedure should also set out how to confirm the identity of those who are unable to communicate.

Identification of staff roles — This should clearly set out the roles and responsibilities and they are often issued by generic staff group. However, staff should also be notified in writing of their entitlement by the IR(ME)R-responsible person for their area.

Pregnancy and breastfeeding — This should provide information of how to obtain the pregnancy and/or breastfeeding status of all female patients deemed to be of childbearing age prior to their exposure. The age range for this is often taken to be 12—55 years of age, and a form confirming the date of the last menstrual period (LMP) is often used.

DRLs — These are compulsory under IR(ME)R and must be audited on a regular basis. Further detail will be given below.

Information on the risks and benefits — Patients must be provided with information around the risks and benefits of the procedure they are undergoing prior to exposure. This can be achieved using posters in reception and waiting areas and by sending out information leaflets with appointment letters.

Reporting of incidents — This should clearly set out the processes for identifying and dealing with these and for how they are to be reported to the appropriate regulatory bodies. Further detail will be given below.

Other procedures which the employer must have in place include those setting out the detail of quality assurance programmes, the implementation of patient dose assessments, and processes for the approval and implementation of research exposures. This will also set out how new acquisition protocols for research exposures are optimised and audited. There will also be procedures for evaluation of exposures, avoidance of unintended exposures, and for non-medical exposures.

DRLs

As stated, DRLs are compulsory under IR(ME)R and advice on how to determine these locally are available from professional bodies, such as IPEM and RCR. There are national DRLs (NDRLs) which are published by Public Health England (PHE)[9] based on national survey results. The NDRL is generally set at the 75th centile of the mean dose obtained from the national survey. Local DRLs are generally below the associated NDRLs and should compare results across different systems for the same examination (i.e., the DRL for a head CT should be consistent across all CT scanners at the site). The image quality of the images produced must be considered during the setting of DRLs, as the limit should be set at a value which is sufficient to obtain images of suitable diagnostic quality whilst maintaining adherence to ALARA. The DRLs should be audited on a regular basis, especially after system upgrades or maintenance.

Incidents

These should be minimised by adherence to the employer's written procedures. However, where they have or are suspected to have occurred, an investigation should be begun immediately. The incidents can be classified as follows:

Accidental exposure — Where the wrong person has been exposed

Unintended exposure — Where the correct person has been exposed but the exposure was greater than intended or the incorrect exposure was carried out. Examples could include use of the wrong modality or imaging of the wrong body part.

Depending on the magnitude of the exposure, these may be deemed to be a *significant accidental or unintended exposure* (SAUE) or a *clinically significant accidental or unintended exposure* (CSAUE). Guidance around the levels

required for these and the reporting procedures are provided by the CQC.[10] The duty of candour applies for all incidents, and the patient should always be appropriately informed.

Carers and Comforters

Carers and comforters are defined explicitly under IR(ME)R 2017 as persons who are exposed whilst supporting or comforting someone undergoing an exposure. This cannot be the case for exposures occurring during their employment, so staff and employees cannot be categorised as carers or comforters. The person exposed must do so knowingly and willingly and therefore must be presented with full information regarding the risks and advice regarding how to minimise their exposure. These are classed as medical exposures and hence must be justified by an appropriate practitioner.

Radionuclide Imaging

All medical uses of radioactive substances now fall under the IR(ME)R 2017 legislation. This now includes radionuclide imaging, or nuclear medicine, which previously fell under the Medicines (Administration of Radioactive Substances) Regulations 1978. This was commonly known as the MARS regulations.

The expert advisory committee for these applications is the Administration of Radioactive Substances Advisory Committee (ARSAC), which was originally founded under the MARS regulations. This body comprises a panel of experts with a membership made up of doctors, physicists, radiopharmacists and radiochemists, and technologists and radiographers with full-time support from a secretariat of staff employed by PHE. They are responsible for advising the licencing authorities as to the suitability of applicants. They also publish a Notes for Guidance[11] (NfG) document which is regularly updated. The information in this document is not mandatory in law but is often defined as being representative of 'good practice', and it contains invaluable information, advice, and data for any institution undertaking radionuclide imaging.

There are two categories of licence required for diagnostic or therapeutic uses of radionuclides and both must be in place for the specific indication before the work commences. Both have a date of issue and expiry (generally 5 years after the date of issue), have a code to identify the specific employer or practitioner, and list the following:

Procedure code — Identifies every procedure for which the licence has been granted

Radionuclide — States the radionuclide licenced for use for that application

Pharmaceutical form — States the pharmaceutical which is being radiolabelled

Indication — States the exact diagnostic or therapeutic purpose for which the given radiopharmaceutical can be used

Research — States whether the specific indication can be used for research purposes under that generic licence. If not, a specific research application must be submitted to use that indication for a research purpose.

The two categories of licence required are:

Employer Licence

This is usually an NHS Trust or Board or a private healthcare firm. They must hold a licence for each site under their ownership where work is carried out with radionuclide sources. On the application, the employer must state who the board level–responsible person is (often the Medical Director), provide a short summary of their IR(ME)R processes, list the MPE staff available and their specific responsibilities, detail their associated equipment, and provide details of their radiopharmaceutical production facilities and staff or their external suppliers.

Practitioner Licence

This must be held by a registered healthcare professional but, in practice, this is always a consultant-level doctor. The holdings on their licence define their scope of practice and they must be appropriately entitled by the employer. The practitioner can list multiple sites and/or employers on their licence but their entitlement and scope of practice must be clear for each. The applicant must detail the specific training they have undertaken and experience they have built up to apply for a licence. The curriculum is detailed in the NfG. Most practitioners are appropriately trained radiologists or physicians, but some may also be oncologists or endocrinologists who have completed appropriate training schemes.

The ARSAC committee are responsible for setting DRLs for each indication and these are also listed in the NfG. There are no DRLs listed for therapeutic applications as the prescribed dose, and hence administered activity is to be determined by the practitioner based on the clinical requirements of the patient. The listed DRLs can be adjusted, generally by body weight or body mass index, at the discretion of the site if sufficient justification can be provided. They will be adjusted downwards for children and smaller adults and upwards for larger or obese patients. This is most often done for myocardial perfusion patients.

All sites involved with medical uses of radionuclides will also require the appropriate permissions from their local environmental protection bodies. These are the Environment Agency (EA) in England, the Scottish Environment Protection Agency (SEPA) in Scotland, Natural Resources Wales (NRW) in Wales, and the Northern Ireland Environment Agency (NIEA) in Northern Ireland. Each site will have licenced holdings for sealed and unsealed radioactive sources, their holdings of waste, and their disposal of waste to the environment. This will also require them to have an entitled and appropriately qualified Radiation Waste Advisor (RWA).

Under the IAEA classification system for sealed radioactive sources, most sources found in hospitals will fall into the level 5, or least hazardous, category. However, many hospitals, especially those with radiotherapy departments providing brachytherapy treatments, will hold sources of sufficient activity to be classed as high-activity sealed sources (HASSs). Information on the activity levels for HASS classification for different radionuclides can be found on the website of the Office for Nuclear Regulation[12] (ONR). HASSs fall under category 2 of the IAEA system and organisations holding them must seek involvement from the local police force and appropriate anti-terrorism advisers to ensure precautions against theft are deemed adequate.

Other legislation which may be encountered by radionuclide imaging departments include the Carriage of Dangerous Goods transport regulations,[13,14] which are enforced by the HSE and ONR. These will be familiar to departments who produce and transport radiopharmaceuticals to other sites but will be encountered by most departments when they purchase new sealed sources for quality-control purposes. It should be highlighted that these rules do not cover the transport of patients, as this falls under IRR regulations.

Transport regulations cover the packaging and labelling of materials in transit and the documentation that is required to accompany them. Advice can be obtained from an appropriately qualified Dangerous Goods Safety Adviser (DGSA). In many cases, the transport companies who are licenced to carry radioactive materials will employ these.

PRACTICAL RADIATION PROTECTION

Engineering Controls

The appropriate design and construction of the physical environment where work with radiation is to be carried out is a fundamental aspect of the protection of staff from exposure. Therefore, radiation protection staff should be involved in the design and planning of new facilities from the earliest stages to ensure that mistakes are not made, as these can be expensive and difficult to correct later in the process. Design considerations can include the placement and opening direction of access doors, positioning of the actual equipment within the room, and the design and placement of shielded workstations for staff within the room. The level of the facility within the building must also be considered to ensure that adequate shielding is provided for staff and facilities occupying spaces on the floors above and below the site.

In addition to the design of facilities, thought must be given to the construction materials and additional shielding requirements to ensure that adequate protection is provided. Depending on the energies of the radiation involved, solid, breeze block–type, block work walls may provide sufficient shielding. These blocks are available in different densities so an appropriate choice can be made. If required, the use of boron concrete can be specified as this increases the effective atomic number and hence shielding of the material. Another common shielding material for construction is the use of different thicknesses of lead bonded to plywood sheets, which can be cut and placed appropriately to deliver the required shielding.

Care must also be taken with any breaks in the shielding, such as pipe or wiring access ducts through walls or ceiling. These should be shielded with lead to maintain the required level of protection. Doors and windows into rooms should also be shielded. This can be achieved using lead glass in windows and using adequate thicknesses of lead sheets within the cores of doors. These will often also have to function as fire doors, so consultation with experts in the implementation of fire safety regulations should be considered. If an RRA deems it necessary, electronic interlock systems can also be fitted to access doors to control entry. Warning signs and lights should be present at any entrance where there is a possibility of exposure upon entry.

Once construction work on new or adapted facilities has finished, the shielding provided should be tested to ensure that it meets the required specifications. This can be achieved using mobile X-ray units or sealed sources of an appropriate energy and activity. These are placed close to the walls and measurements are taken outside the room using appropriate radiation detectors. Calculations can then be made of the shielding provided and this can be compared to the specified values.

Dosimeters

The employer will provide staff with dosimeters to be worn if they are regularly working with radiation. The most common of these are film-based body badges to monitor whole-body exposure. These should be worn on the body at all times and will be replaced regularly with the interval being determined by the likelihood of exposure to significant radiation doses. For example, staff in nuclear medicine will often have their badges changed monthly whereas staff in dental practices using only low-dose dental X-rays may only have theirs replaced at two- or three-month intervals.

For certain staff groups, the film badges may be complemented by additional thermoluminescent dosimeters (TLD) to monitor eye or extremity doses. Staff likely to be exposed to the highest dose rates may also be supplied with electronic personal dosimeters (EPDs), as these allow real-time monitoring of exposure and may provide audible warnings of dose rate to highlight to staff when they are at greatest risk.

Film Badge

The film badge consists of a photographic film, which records the exposure the wearer is subject to, and a holder, which will contain sections with differing attenuation properties to allow estimation of the energies of the incident radiation. Metal foils and metals such as copper, aluminium, and lead are often used as the attenuating materials along with the plastic body of the badge itself. Some may contain film with different emulsions to optimise the response to high and low doses of radiation such that the badge provides accurate responses at the low doses generally encountered but can also cope accurately with an unintended sudden exposure to a high dose.

TLDs

The most common TLDs used in the healthcare environment are typically chips of lithium fluoride within a plastic holder. Energy imparted from the incident radiation is stored within the crystalline lattice of the lithium fluoride until sufficient heat is applied to liberate the energy as visible light. Thus, once the TLD has been exposed, it will store the information until it is placed in a specialised reader to release the light. The amount of light given off is directly proportional to the dose of radiation to which the crystal was exposed. The reader consists of a small oven which will heat the crystal to the required temperature, typically over 200 °C, and a light detector and processor which measures and records the resulting light output.

For measurement of extremity doses, TLDs can be attached to the frame of a pair of glasses or goggles to measure eye dose or placed in rings or finger stalls to measure finger doses. The stalls fit over the tip of the finger and provide the best estimate of the dose to the finger. However, these can be difficult for staff to wear as they interfere with dexterity, they are prone to being quite fragile and break frequently, and they may not comply with local hand hygiene regulations. For these reasons, finger rings are often worn on the inside surface of the base of a finger and a correction factor is applied to the measurements to approximate the dose at the tip of the finger. However, these may not provide sufficient accuracy to meet regulatory requirements due to uncertainty in calculation of the correction factors. TLD finger rings are commonly worn by staff in nuclear medicine and radiopharmacy who are involved in the production and manipulation of radiopharmaceuticals.

EPDs

EPDs use semiconductor devices to measure and record incident dose rates, mostly being used in areas where these are likely to be highest. A digital readout can display the incident dose rate and/or the cumulative dose since the device was last reset. This often occurs when the wearer starts their shift or commences a task where the exposure is likely to be high. As mentioned, these can also provide audible warnings of the incident dose rate or when the cumulative dose reaches a defined threshold. Some EPDs available now can be networked or connected via Bluetooth or similar technologies to allow remote recording of all exposures.

Personal Protective Equipment (PPE)

The PPE provided for staff will include disposable gloves and aprons, especially for staff working with unsealed radioactive sources, although many staff will wear these routinely as part of infection control measures. Staff working in higher dose-rate areas may have lead aprons available to reduce body dose. These can be provided in different thicknesses of lead depending upon the likely dose rates but can be prohibitively heavy for some staff in the higher thicknesses. Aprons containing other materials such as tin have been developed to try and overcome weight issues.

Care must also be taken that the use of shielded aprons does not actually increase the exposure to the wearer. In some areas where the energy of the incident radiation is higher, such as nuclear medicine, the aprons may just precipitate secondary scatter, which is at energies which are more easily absorbed by the wearer's body. Staff working in high dose-rate areas, such as interventional theatres, may also wear lead shields for the thyroid and protective lead glass goggles to reduce eye doses.

Staff working in areas with sealed and unsealed radioactive sources may also wear disposable foot covers in addition to the aprons and gloves used routinely. These mitigate the potential of any contamination or spills being spread from the work area if they are removed upon exit

from the area and disposed of appropriately. Disposable sleeves may also be worn to protect exposed skin on the arms from spills or contamination to minimise skin doses. These are especially important where alpha- or beta-emitting radionuclides are being used.

Patient Dosimetry

The dose and risk to the patient can be minimised by adherence to the recommendations and requirements of the IRR and IR(ME)R regulations. This includes having appropriately trained staff, equipment which undergoes regular and appropriate quality control, and robust processes for dose optimisation, justification, and reporting of examinations. Avoidance of having to repeat exposures to obtain clinically useful images of sufficient image quality is one of the easiest ways to ensure patient doses are minimised.

Most radiology or nuclear medicine departments will display posters in their receptions and waiting rooms which provide the patients with information around the relative risks of the studies they are about to undergo. They will also display posters asking any patients who suspect they may be pregnant to inform a member of staff prior to their test such that informed decisions can be made around whether the examination should proceed. There are now readily available, nationally developed posters for these purposes which can help to ensure compliance with the regulatory requirements.

As mentioned earlier, the effective dose to a patient cannot be directly measured and can only be approximated using conversions from measured parameters such as entrance surface dose and DAP for planar X-ray examinations. As IR(ME)R requires all patient exposures to be ALARP, most modern radiological imaging equipment now provides a record of one of these parameters for all exposures which can be stored or sent to picture archiving and communication systems (PACS) or radiology systems as a dose report. These allow calculation of effective doses to the patient which can be compared to local or national DRLs and allow regular auditing to take place.

The conversion factors for calculation of effective doses are generally highest for the more radiosensitive organs in the abdomen and chest and lowest for the head and limbs. There may also be variations depending on the projection of the image being obtained relative to the positioning of the organ. For example, the conversion factor for the stomach will be higher for an anterior projection than a posterior projection due to the anterior location of the stomach within the abdomen. The conversion factors for DAP typically range between 0.05 and 0.25 $mSv/mGycm^2$ but can be higher for the most radiosensitive tissues.

In CT, the effective dose depends not on the area of the patient exposed, as in a planar X-ray, but on the volume of the patient imaged, which depends on the scan length. Therefore, the measured parameter which is often quoted is the dose length product (DLP) in mGycm. This is derived from the CT dose index (CTDI) multiplied by the length of the scan in centimetres. The CTDI is measured in a tissue-equivalent phantom or using Monte Carlo—based computer simulations from CT data to give a dose in Gy. The conversion factors for DLP range between 0.002 mSv/mGycm for a CT scan of the head and 0.015 mSv/mGycm for a scan of the abdomen and pelvis.

Table 2.7 lists the effective doses for a wide range of common radiological examinations. Given that the average yearly dose in the UK from background radiation is 2.7 mSv, this demonstrates that the examinations listed give a dose equivalent to a few hours to a few years of background exposure.

The recorded doses for certain examinations also allow regular dose audits to be carried out, as required by IR(ME)R. These allow comparison of the dose for a particular examination with the appropriate local and national DRLs and for assessment of the variation in doses for a particular examination between different imaging systems. It should be noted that individual patient doses may exceed local or national DRLs, especially for larger patients or reasons of specific pathology. Therefore, it is the average dose over a sufficiently large number of patients which should be used for comparisons.

TABLE 2.7 Approximate Effective Doses from a Range of Common Radiological Examinations

Study	Approximate Effective Dose (mSv)
CT head and neck	1.2
CT brain — repeated with and without contrast	3.2
CT chest	6.1
CT coronary angiography	8.7
CT spine	8.8
CT abdomen and pelvis	7.7
CT abdomen and pelvis — repeated with and without contrast	15.4
CT colonoscopy	6.0
Barium enema	6.0
Chest X-ray	0.1
Lumbar spine X-ray	1.4
Hand X-ray	0.001
Dental X-ray	0.005
Dental panoramic X-ray (OPT)	0.025
Mammogram	0.25
DEXA bone densitometry scan	0.001
Nuclear medicine bone scan — whole body	2.9
Nuclear medicine cerebral perfusion scan	7.0
Nuclear medicine MAG3 renogram	0.7
Nuclear medicine FDG PET scan*	7.6

*This is the dose purely from the radiopharmaceutical component of the exam. The dose from the CT component will vary depending on the quality and complexity of the CT required. CT, computed tomography; DEXA, dual-energy X-ray absorptiometry; FDG, fluorodeoxyglucose; OPT, optical projection tomography; PET, positron emission tomography.

REFERENCES

1. Valentin J. Low-dose extrapolation of radiation-related cancer risk. *Ann ICRP*. 2005;35:1—140.
2. ICRP. 1990 Recommendations of the international commission on radiological protection. *Ann ICRP*. 1991;21:1—201.
3. UK Statutory Instruments. *The Ionising Radiation (Medical Exposure) Regulations 2017*; 2017 [Online]. Available at: https://www.legislation.gov.uk/uksi/2017/1322/contents/made. (Accessed on: 05 May 2022).
4. UK Statutory Instruments. *The Ionising Radiations Regulations 2017*; 2017 [Online]. Available at: https://www.legislation.gov.uk/uksi/2017/1075/contents/made. (Accessed on: 05 May 2022).
5. Health and Safety Executive. *Working with Ionising Radiation: Ionising Radiations Regulations 2017: Approved Code of Practice and Guidance*. 2nd ed. Norwich, UK: The Stationery Office; 2018.
6. Saunderson JR, others. *Medical and Dental Guidance Notes: A Good Practice Guide on All Aspects of Ionising Radiation Protection in the Clinical Environment*. 10th ed. York, UK: IPEM; 2002.
7. Northern Ireland Statutory Rules. *The Ionising Radiation (Medical Exposure) Regulations Northern Ireland 2018*; 2018. Available at: https://www.legislation.gov.uk/nisr/2018/17/contents/made. (Accessed on: 05 May 2022).
8. Department of Health and Social Care. *Guidance to the Ionising Radiation (Medical Exposure) Regulations 2017*; 2018 [Online]. Available at: https://assets.publishing.service.gov.uk/government/uploads/system/uploads/attachment_data/file/720282/guidance-to-the-ionising-radiation-medical-exposure-regulations-2017.pdf. (Accessed on: 05 May 2022).
9. Public Health England. *National Diagnostic Reference Levels (NDRLs) from 19 August 2019*; 2019. Available at: https://www.gov.uk/government/publications/diagnostic-radiology-national-diagnostic-reference-levels-ndrls/ndrl. (Accessed on: 05 May 2022).
10. Care Quality Commission. *SAUE: Criteria for Making a Notification*; 2020 [Online]. Available at: https://cqc.org.uk/

guidance-providers/ionising-radiation/saue-criteria-making-notification. (Accessed on: 05 May 2022).

11. Administration of Radioactive Substances Advisory Committee. *Notes for Guidance on the Clinical Administration of Radiopharmaceuticals and Use of Sealed Radioactive Sources*; 2021 [Online]. Available at: https://assets.publishing.service.gov.uk/government/uploads/system/uploads/attachment_data/file/961343/ARSAC_NfG_Feb2021.pdf. (Accessed on: 05 May 2022).

12. Office for Nuclear Regulation. *High-Activity Sealed Radioactive Sources (HASS) on Nuclear Licensed Sites*; 2020 [Online].

Available at: https://www.onr.org.uk/hass.htm. (Accessed on: 05 May 2022).

13. UK Statutory Instruments. *The Carriage of Dangerous Goods and Use of Transportable Pressure Equipment Regulations 2009*; 2009 [Online]. Available at: https://www.legislation.gov.uk/uksi/2009/1348/contents/made. (Accessed on: 05 May 2022).

14. Statutory Instruments. *Radioactive Substances: The Carriage of Dangerous Goods (Amendment) Regulations 2019*; 2019 [Online]. Available at: https://www.legislation.gov.uk/uksi/2019/598/pdfs/uksi_20190598_en.pdf. (Accessed on: 05 May 2022).

X-Ray Imaging

CHAPTER CONTENTS

Harnessing the X-ray has yielded various imaging possibilities. This chapter will cover general radiography, mammography, and fluoroscopy. The original analogue systems have been superseded and replaced by digital systems. Some information about analogue systems is included in this chapter, only to demonstrate the underlying concepts and principles.

X-RAY TUBE AND X-RAY BEAM

X-rays are produced when fast-moving electrons undergo interaction with a metal target. The kinetic energy of the electrons is converted to X-rays ($\sim$1%) and heat ($\sim$99%).

The following are further considerations of the X-ray tube mentioned in the first chapter.

Cathode — This is constructed of a tungsten coil/filament (0.1–0.5 mm). It has a high melting point (3,422 °C) which enables thermionic emission. This requires heating the filament to >2200 °C, allowing electrons to absorb enough kinetic energy to escape the wire surface.

Focussing cup — This is used to minimise electron spread. It also causes the electron stream to converge on a limited area of the target anode. The cup must have a high heat tolerance and a low thermionic emission potential. It is negatively charged to direct electrons to the anode. The cup can be of different sizes to yield different focal spot sizes.

Anode — The anode is composed of a tungsten/rhenium alloy target. Rhenium is used for ductility (to prevent cracking). The surface of the target is smooth and flat at production. After repeated use, it can suffer from pitting (small pits and holes in the surface). The surface of the anode is angled with the target angle, usually at 7–20°. By using a smaller angle, a narrower X-ray spectrum and smaller field are produced. The core of the anode is composed of molybdenum or graphite. This core facilitates heat conduction to prevent damage to the metal bearings. The core is lubricated with silver which has no effect on heat transfer.

The anode may be stationary or rotating. Stationary anodes are used in dental radiology. A rotating anode is used for most X-ray applications.

Heating is a limiting factor in X-ray production. Excessive rises in temperature may melt component parts. To minimise geometric and movement unsharpness, the focal spot and exposure time should be as small as possible. The focal spot size is shown in Fig. 3.1. There are two spots. The first is the actual focal spot, which is the area over which heat is produced, and which determines the tube rating. The second is the effective focal spot, which indicates the beam area exiting the tube. The exposure time should also be as short as possible, but this leads to high-input milliamperage on a very small target (and increases heat production).

The rotating anode is used to spread the produced heat over a larger area. It results in a focal track rather than spot (ring T in Fig. 3.1C). It is based on an induction motor-driven copper rotor, which rotates at 3000 rpm. Anode cooling is achieved through the following steps. The first step is for heat produced on the focal track to be conducted to the anode disk. This heat is then radiated to the insulating oil around the rotor. The anode assembly is blackened to encourage heat radiation. The rate of heat loss is proportional to temperature[4] (in kelvin).

The heat rating reflects the allowable *milliamperage* per particular kV values (kV × mA, with units in joules). This rating decreases based on the following factors:

- Longer exposure time
- Increased kV
- Reduced rotation

The rating increases based on the following factors:

- Increased effective focal spot size
- Increased anode diameter (increased focal track size)
- Rotating anode vs stationary
- Increased rotation speed

Uniformity of the beam: An X-ray tube emits some X-rays in every direction, necessitating lead shielding inside the tube housing to protect the patient and staff from unnecessary exposure. A collimator system is used to adjust the beam to the required size. The collimator system comprises two sets of parallel blades made of high-attenuation material that can be driven into the beam to define the required (rectangular) area.

The useful beam is taken off where it is most intense, in a direction perpendicular to the electron stream. The central ray (Fig. 3.2, line B) emerges at right angles to the tube axis from the centre of the focal spot. It is usually pointed towards the centre of the area of interest in the body.

The maximum size of the useful beam is determined by angle θ of the anode. In practice, it is narrower than suggested because of the *heel effect*. As indicated in Fig. 3.2, most of the electrons penetrate a few micrometres into the target before being stopped by a nucleus. On their way out, the X-rays are attenuated and filtered by the target material. X-rays travelling towards the anode edge of the field (line A) have more target material to cross and so are attenuated more than those travelling towards the cathode edge (line C). The intensity of the beam decreases across the field, and this is most apparent from B to A. The steeper the target, the greater the heel effect.

The heel effect, being gradual, is generally not noticeable even on the largest detector. Where the patient's thickness varies considerably across the field, advantage may be taken of the heel effect by positioning the patient with the thicker or denser part towards the cathode of the tube where the exit beam is more intense (in mammography).

The intensity of the beam decreases somewhat either side of the central ray, in a direction perpendicular to AC (i.e., parallel to the tube axis), because of the inverse square law, the X-rays at the edges having further to travel.

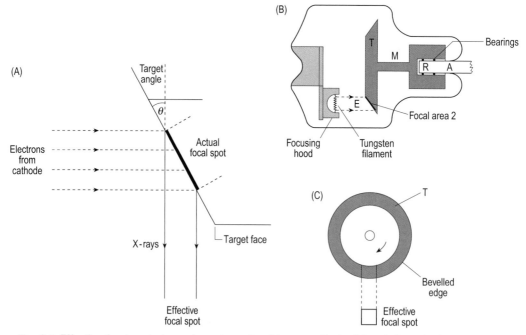

Fig. 3.1 Effective focal spot size and anode angle with perpendicular (a) and through plane views (c). *E*, electron beam; *T*, anode disk; *M,* molybdenum stem; *R,* rotor; *A,* axle sealed in the glass envelope.

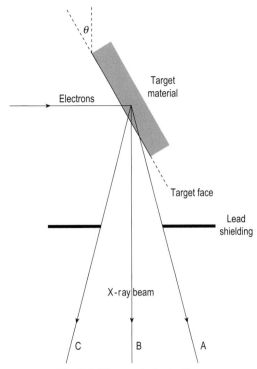

Fig. 3.2 The anode heel effect.

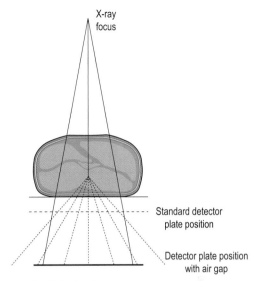

Fig. 3.3 An air gap used to reduce scatter.

Scatter Rejection

Primary radiation reflects the information about the intervening object along a direct path from source to detector. The information is based on the intensity, governed by (from Chapter 1): $I = I_0 e^{-\mu d}$

Scattered radiation is radiation that obscures information about the imaged object (artificially increases intensity). The amount of scattered radiation (S) reaching a detector is usually several times that of the primary radiation (P). Scatter reduces image contrast by a factor of $[1 + S/P]$, up to 10 times. To combat scatter, there are several reduction and improvement strategies.

- Reduce the volume of the irradiated tissue via collimation of field area
- Compress the tissue to reduce the height of the tissue irradiated
- Reduced kV to increase the photoelectric absorption vs Compton scatter
- Air gap — The image plate is moved away from the patient. This reduces the scatter that hits the image detector plate (see Fig. 3.3). This does, however, produce a magnified image. As the distance is increased, increased kV or mA is required to maintain photon flux
- Grid (see below)

The grid consists of lead strips 50–70 μm wide. Between each strip is interspace material, which is of low attenuation, usually carbon fibre. The line density is usually 30–80 grid lines/cm (typically 40 grid lines/cm). Low frequency is considered 40–50 grid lines/cm, 50–60 grid lines/cm is medium frequency, and >60 grid lines/cm is high frequency. A parallel/unfocussed grid is shown in Fig. 3.4, with each lead strip parallel to each other. Scattered radiation outside the acceptance angle θ is absorbed by the strips of lead.

The grid ratio represents the depth:width (d:w in Fig. 3.4). The grid ratio is usually at least 8:1, but it can be up to 16:1.

A focussed grid (see Fig. 3.5) uses lead strips that are tilted progressively to the point source. The use of a focussed grid is more defined with specific operational tolerances, which increase depending on grid ratio. There is a defined anode-grid distance. The grid must be accurately centred to the anode. The grid cannot be tilted.

A moving grid is a method used to blur out grid lines on the detector. It is for low-frequency grids. The grid moves parallel to the detector plane during exposure of the image, causing the grid lines to be blurred.

The contrast improvement factor represents the ratio of contrast with a grid to that without a grid, with a value usually between 2 and 4.

The grid factor represents the increased mA required to achieve the same exposure when using a grid, with values of 3–5.

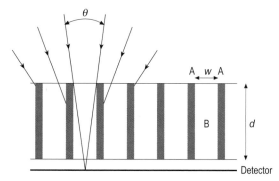

Fig. 3.4 Detailed construction of a parallel anti-scatter grid. *W*, gap between lead strips; *A*, thickness of lead strip; *B*, interspace material; *d*, height of grid.

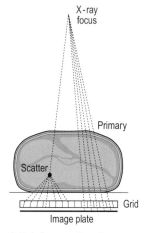

Fig. 3.5 A focussed anti-scatter grid.

$$\frac{\text{Exposure necessary with grid}}{\text{Exposure necessary without grid}}$$

The signal-to-noise improvement factor is represented by $\sqrt{(\text{Grid factor})}$.

Grid selectivity indicates the ability of a grid to transmit primary radiation and absorb scattered radiation.

$$\frac{\text{Fraction of primary radiation transmitted}}{\text{Fracture of scattered radiation transmitted}}$$

The fraction of primary radiation transmitted can be calculated from the ratio of $w : (w+A)$ from Fig. 3.4. The

fraction of scattered radiation transmitted depends on the grid ratio and kV. The range is usually 6–12.

X-Ray Room

Room

The room used for the X-ray machine must be specially designed. The whole room is lead lined to prevent irradiation of surrounding rooms. An overview of a typical room is shown in Figs. 3.6 and 3.7.

The exam area contains several components. There is an adjustable patient table with a built-in digital detector. There is a wall-mounted detector apparatus with a built-in digital detector. This is connected to the control room computer via cables. There is a ceiling-mounted X-ray source, which can be moved to operate with the table or wall-mounted detectors. When the radiograph is to be obtained, the room is sealed to prevent any scattered radiation escaping the room.

The control area is behind a lead-shielded window, in which the equipment controls and process computers are kept. The acquisition of the radiograph is supervised from this area.

Portable

Some patients are too ill to travel to the X-ray room. Portable devices are required to image these patients (see Fig. 3.8). These devices contain everything needed for image acquisition, processing, storage, and subsequent transmission to the picture archiving and communication system (PACS).

Computed Radiography (CR)

These systems are functional with conventional analogue X-ray equipment. They allow for the transition from film-screen radiography to digital output to be cheaper and more straightforward for departments with older hardware.

This system uses a storage cassette, which is similar to that used in conventional analogue X-ray equipment. It contains a photostimulable phosphor plate to store energy from the incident X-rays. The plate requires light input to release the trapped energy. The light used is proportional to the X-ray intensity. The plate is commonly composed of barium fluorohalide doped with europium (BaFX:Eu; X – halide; usually 85:15 combination of bromide and iodide), as a 0.3-mm layer of powdered material on a containing plate. A surface coat protects the phosphor from physical damage, and the plate is contained in a light-tight cassette.

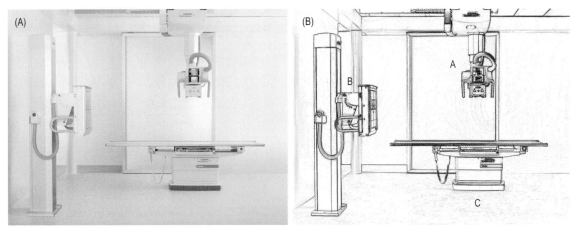

Fig. 3.6 (A) Conventional X-ray room; (B) labelled. *A*, ceiling-mounted X-ray source; *B*, wall-mounted detector apparatus; *C*, adjustable patient table with under table detector plate. (Credit Siemens Healthcare Ltd.)

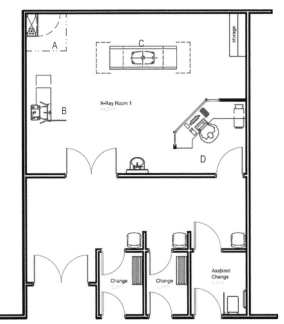

Fig. 3.7 Room layout. *A*, Ceiling-mounted X-ray source; *B*, wall-mounted detector apparatus; *C*, adjustable patient table with under table detector plate; *D*, control area. (Credit Siemens Healthcare Ltd.)

A CR reader is used to retrieve the radiographic image. An overview of the system is shown in Fig. 3.9. In the reader, the plate is removed from the cassette and scanned with a laser beam. Red laser light is used as most phosphors release blue light. A rotating mirror is used for scanning.

Photomultiplier tubes measure the light intensity emitted from each scanned section of the plate, in a line-by-line image extraction process. The photomultiplier tubes amplify the recorded signal, which is then converted to electronic signal using an analogue-to-digital converter. The plate image is then erased afterwards by exposing the plate to a bright light source. The overall process takes 30–45 seconds.

Image processing—The photostimulable phosphors have a very wide dynamic range (10,000:1). There would be very limited contrast if white is set to 1, and black to 10,000 (see Fig. 3.10), with most of the acquired radiographic images appearing mostly grey. The response of the system is linear, compared to the older film-screen system which had a characteristic curve. Some initial image processing is performed before export to PACS. This first step is to ignore signals from outside the collimated area. The second step is histogram analysis of the distribution of light intensities in the collimated area. The histogram is processed to reject extremes of high and low signals (see Fig. 3.11). The third step involves applying a gradation curve to optimise readability. Further processing such as edge enhancement of noise reduction can be performed before distribution to PACS.

Image Quality

Spatial resolution — The spatial resolution of CR is less than analogue film-screen radiography. The main limiting factor is the pixel size, which varies between plates. Pixel sizes of ~90 μm are used for small plates: there are 2000×2670 pixels in 18×24 cm^2, yielding 5.5 lp/mm.

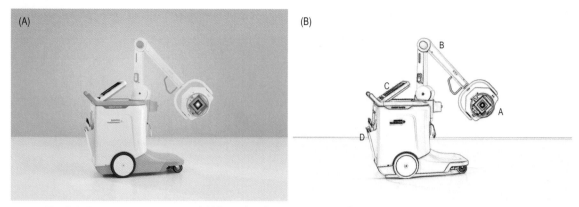

Fig. 3.8 Portable X-ray machine. *A*, X-Ray tube; *B*, adjustable arm; *C*, control interface; *D*, detector storage for transport. (Credit Siemens Healthcare Ltd.)

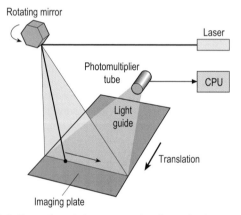

Fig. 3.9 Formation of the computed radiography image using a scanned laser beam. *CPU*, central processing unit.

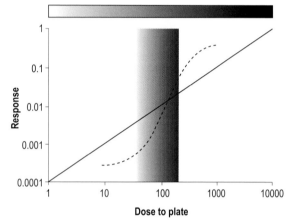

Fig. 3.10 Relation between signal from a computed radiography plate and dose to the plate. For comparison, the characteristic curve of a film-screen system is shown (dashed line).

These are used for peripheral imaging. Pixels sizes of $\sim$140 µm are used for larger plates, with 2500 × 3070 pixels in 35 × 43 cm^2, yielding 3.5 lp/mm. These are used for chest or abdominal imaging ($\sim$50 µm for mammography). In comparison, film-screen resolution is 8–12 lp/mm.

The laser reading stage affects the resolution as there is inherent scatter in the phosphor layer. A thinner phosphor layer decreases scatter and improves spatial resolution. Smaller phosphor crystal size also improves spatial resolution.

Contrast — Defined by histogram analysis and gradation curve, as the dose-response is linear. There is no characteristic curve as in film-screen radiography.

Detector dose indicators (DDIs) — These are assurance mechanisms to measure doses given to patients. These are present to keep incident doses as low as reasonably

practicable. DDIs are manufacturer dependent and need to be validated according to local departmental diagnostic reference levels (DRLs).

Artefacts

Image acquisition stage:
- Moiré pattern — interference between grid and laser scan lines. Grids with >60 lines/cm should be used
- Ghost artefact — imaging plate was not erased after previous use
- Fading of image — delay in acquisition and processing
- Light bulb effect — backscattered radiation
- Overexposure or underexposure — failure of autoranging software

- Cracks or focal radiopacities — fault with imaging plate or dust

Image processing:

- Linear radiopaque or radiolucent lines — indicate a malfunctioning plate reader

Digital Radiography (DR)

The efficiency of an X-ray detector system is based on the detective quantum efficiency (DQE). This indicates the

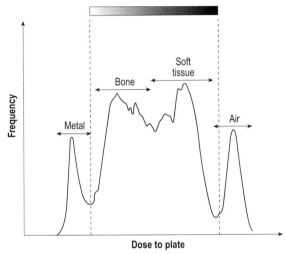

Fig. 3.11 Distribution of signals from the computed radiography plate as a function of dose.

efficiency of photon detection and the effects of added noise to the detected signal. A perfect system with full photon detection and no noise yields a DQE of 100%. CR systems can achieve a DQE of ~30%. DR systems can achieve ~65%.

DR comes in two classes: direct and indirect conversion. A brief graphical comparison between incident X-ray photon and output electrical signal is shown in Fig. 3.12.

Direct conversion — This process directly converts incident X-ray photons to an electronic signal.

An overview of the method using amorphous selenium is shown in Fig. 3.13. The first layer is an electrode, which has a small positive charge applied prior to use. The second layer is that of the photoconductor, which absorbs X-ray photons. Electrons are released by the selenium dependent upon interaction with an X-ray. The released electrons migrate to the surface electrode. Positive charge is drawn to the charge collecting electrode (with minimal lateral diffusion) and stored in a storage capacitor in the thin-flat panel transistor (TFT) layer. This charge forms the latent radiographic image. The processing and readout of these stored charges is controlled by gating the switches of the TFT layer.

TFT layer — This is an array of very small detector elements (DELs). Each element contains a few components (see Fig. 3.14):

- Pixel or capture element — detects electrical signals
- Storage capacitor — stores the electric charge produced by the capture element

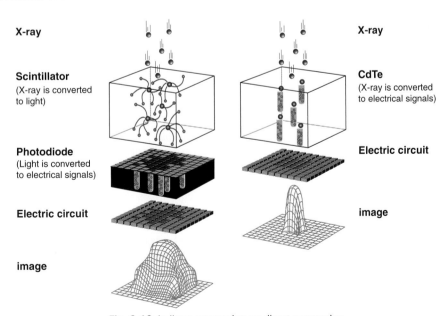

Fig. 3.12 Indirect conversion vs direct conversion.

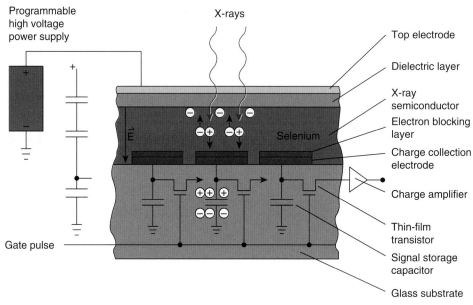

Fig. 3.13 Cross-section of an amorphous selenium (a-Se) detector for direct digital radiography. *TFT,* thin-film transistor.

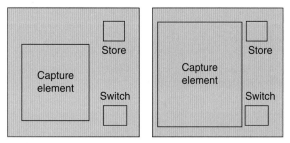

Fig. 3.14 Detector element layout, demonstrating different fill factors.

- Switch — governs the release of the electric charge in the storage capacitor
- The fill factor reflects the percentage area of the overall DEL area taken up by the capture element

Another method for direct conversion uses a charge-coupled device (CCD). These devices are widely used in modern visual equipment, like camcorders and digital cameras. These are solid-state devices. Each is fast, sensitive, and with minimal burn-in. They also have excellent thermal, electrical, and magnetic stability.

CCDs operate using semiconductor capacitors with photosensitive elements. Here, the photon creates an electron-hole pair. The released electrons accumulate in a potential well. The charge yielded by this potential well is indicative of the incident radiation dose.

CCDs have pixel detectors with image capture and frame storage regions. The image capture regions integrate charge from the photosensitive element. The charge is integrated over a set period to capture an image. The frame rate is usually 25 Hz. The charge is then transferred to the frame storage region at a rate determined by the pixel clock. This charge is used to generate a voltage which is then digitised to greyscale to form the output image. Whilst this output image is read for display, the image capture region is concurrently acquiring a new image.

There are three modes of acquisition for a CCD:
1. Full frame — The entire image area is active. This mode is slow and requires mechanical shuttering during the read-out phase.
2. Frame transfer — Half of the light-sensitive silicon area is shielded at a time. The output image is transferred from the active to shielded area for read-out. This mode needs twice the area of silicon.
3. Interline transfer — Every other line is shielded. This mode is very fast, but half as efficient.

Indirect conversion: This process first converts X-ray photons to light photons, and then the light photons are converted to electric signal. An overview of the system is shown in Fig. 3.15. The initial conversion occurs in the scintillator layer and is achieved with a phosphor (e.g., caesium iodide or gadolinium oxysulphide). The

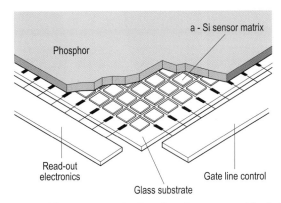

Fig. 3.15 The structure of a flat plate detector used for indirect digital radiography. *a-Si*, amorphous silicon.

phosphor crystals are aligned perpendicular to the detector surface. This alignment causes any internal reflections to be directed towards the detector surface. As the amount of scatter is reduced by this, a thick layer may be used (increases detection efficiency). In the photodiode layer, light photons are converted to electronic signal. This layer is composed of hydrogenated amorphous silicon. Below the photodiode is the TFT array, like the one used in direct conversion.

Artefacts in DR

- Detector drops — These are white or black artefacts after individual pixels or electronics are damaged. The system can interpolate surrounding pixel information to correct for this ('pixel calibration')
- Backscatter — Backscattered radiation from detector electronics visible on image
- Image saturation — Loss of information when the processing algorithm dynamic range is exceeded
- Detector offset correction failure or ghost image — Previous image was not cleared
- Detector calibration limitation — Image artefacts when the exposure exceeds calibration conditions; faulty calibration causes artefact, usually excessively low or high density
- Grid-line suppression failure — Software post-processing failure
- Aliasing/Moiré pattern — caused by low-frequency antiscatter grids; the high-contrast signal is still resolvable by the detector

Image Processing

Greyscale processing — This method of image processing is based on the image histogram. The histogram demonstrates graphically the number of pixels for each allotted brightness level. Alterations to the histogram allow for brightness and contrast manipulation, as well as compressing the range of values displayed. This can also improve the balance of the image by reducing focal intensities.

Windowing — window width alters the image contrast, whilst the window alters the image brightness.

Look-up table (LUT) — Similar to the characteristic curve of conventional film radiography. Each modality (X-ray, computed tomography, magnetic resonance imaging, ultrasonography) and body part have a specific LUT to maximise contrast and brightness. Each pixel value is altered to enhance the displayed image.

Auto-ranging — This is an automated analysis of the image histogram. It excludes very high and low values which would otherwise adversely affect the image contrast and brightness. The remainder of the image histogram is normalised to maximise image display.

Fig. 3.16 demonstrates images of a left ankle with various manipulations of the histogram performed on a PACS workstation:

- A — standard post-processed image. Full visibility of soft tissues and bone
- B — high pixel values only. Every value below 2972 is represented as black
- C — every pixel above 1084 is represented as white
- D — every pixel above 2051 is represented as white
- E — every pixel below 2033 is represented as black
- F — very narrow window [2961 3022], causing most values to be black or white
- G — every pixel above 3012 is represented as white
- H — every pixel below 1080 is represented as black
- I — the window of the histogram [−17036 21188], has been far extended from the acquired pixel values [0 4095], thus causing all the acquired data to be in a very limited region of the histogram window. As such, the image appears mostly grey with little contrast between the various pixels

Filtering — Another processing method is to filter the image in the spatial location and frequency domains. This can be achieved through several methods:

- Convolution — A mathematical process involving a predefined kernel (a small matrix operator with specific purpose; e.g., edge detection, blurring, sharpening). This process adds weighted values of each surrounding pixel to the original.
- Low-pass filtering to smooth the image — This is a technique in which the greyscale value stored in each pixel is increased by a proportion of the value of the neighbouring pixels and the resultant value is averaged. The effect is to smooth the final image, but it will blur small details or edges.

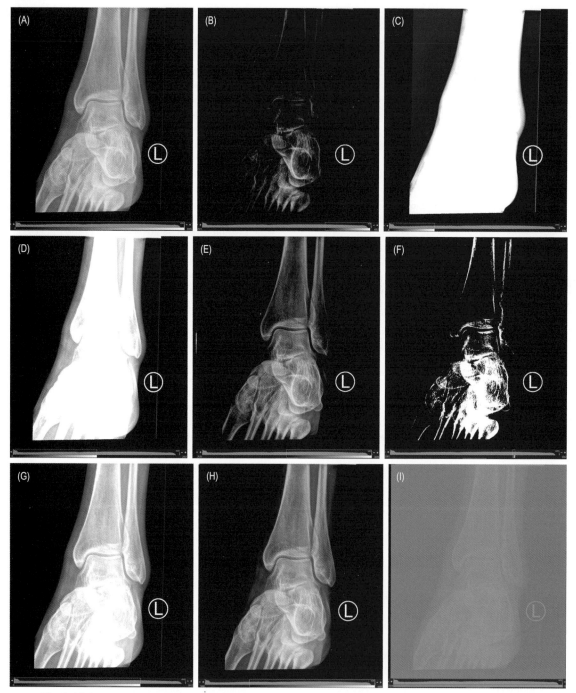

Fig. 3.16 Images of a left ankle after different manipulations of the histogram. The acquired data is present in the grey graph at the bottom. The white box indicates the range of the histogram used, with the lower and upper limits of each histogram in the bottom left and right of each image.

- High-pass filtering for edge enhancement — A high-pass filter adds in a proportion of the difference between the greyscale value of the pixel and that of its neighbours. The effect is to exaggerate the contrast at the boundary between structures, thus making the structures more visible. However, the process also serves to increase noise. It may generate false structures in the image when a high level of filtering is applied.
- Spatial feature enhancement.

Temporal averaging — using multiple sets of the same image acquired over time to reduce noise in the image.

Digital Image Quality

Sampling — The *Nyquist* criterion states that the signal must be sampled *at least twice in every cycle or period*, or that the sampling frequency must be at least twice the highest frequency present in the signal. Otherwise, high-frequency signals will erroneously be recorded as low, referred to as *aliasing*. The maximum signal frequency that can be accurately sampled is called the Nyquist frequency and is equal to half of the sampling frequency. Fig. 3.17A shows a sine wave (solid curve) that is sampled four times in three cycles. The samples, shown by the squares, are interpreted by the imaging system as a wave (dashed curve) of much lower frequency. Sampling six times in the same period, as in Fig. 3.17B, preserves the correct frequency.

Modulation transfer function (MTF) — This represents the fidelity with which an imaging system records spatial frequency. Limits to resolution are intrinsic to the imaging modality and equipment. In particular, sharp edges are not perfectly represented but suffer a certain degree of blurring. Fig. 3.18 shows the profile of a grid pattern produced by a test object. Fig. 3.18A represents a low spatial frequency (i.e., widely spaced detail) in which blurring is not sufficient to prevent the modulation of the output signal profile from matching the modulation present in the object. Modulation here represents the difference between the maximum and minimum amplitude as a proportion of the average signal. As the spatial frequency is progressively increased in Figs. 3.18B and C, the blurring reduces the output modulation such that with the addition of noise it would become impossible to visualise detail at the higher spatial frequencies. The MTF represents the ratio of the output and input modulation. The MTF varies with spatial

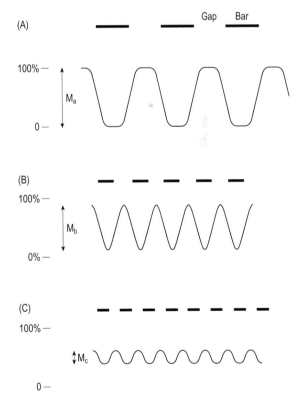

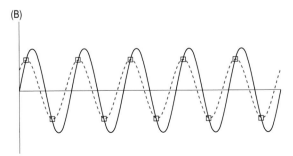

Fig. 3.17 The dashed waveforms represent those recorded. (A) Aliasing produces a different waveform than the true waveform due to under-sampling. (B) The sampling satisfies the Nyquist criterion, and the true waveform is recorded.

Fig. 3.18 The output signal behind a grid pattern, showing reduction in modulation caused by blurring as spatial frequency increases.

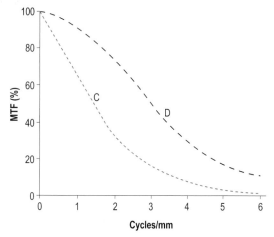

Fig. 3.19 Modulation transfer function (MTF) as a function of spatial frequency for various radiographic systems. *C,* computed radiography; *D,* direct digital radiography.

frequency, generally reducing progressively from 100% at low spatial frequencies (perfect system) towards zero at higher frequencies. MTF as a function of spatial frequency is shown in Fig. 3.19 for CR and DR imaging systems. A CR system is limited by the phosphor (the laser light used to read the signal is scattered within). An indirect DR system is also limited by the phosphor layer, but not to the same degree as a CR system. A direct DR system is limited by pixel size.

The DQE of the system is defined as SNR^2_{out}/SNR^2_{in}, where SNR is the signal-to-noise ratio. It is a common way to compare two systems by quoting a single figure such as the spatial frequency at which the MTF is 10%.

The quantum sink is the stage which degrades overall DQE of an imaging system, caused by noise in a finite number of quanta.

Contrast

This encompasses the ability to distinguish between regions of an image (see Fig. 3.20). Accordingly, subject contrast C depends on the thickness t of the structure and the difference in linear attenuation coefficients, μ_1 and μ_2, of the tissues involved.

$$\text{Contrast } \alpha \ (\mu_1 - \mu_2)$$

Improved contrast is facilitated by

- Thicker structure
- Greater difference in attenuation coefficients

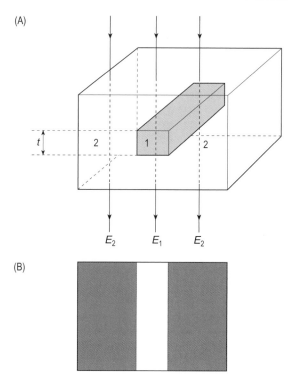

Fig. 3.20 Primary contrast produced (A) on imaging a structure (1, bone) that is surrounded by a uniform block of another material (2, soft tissue); and (B) a representation of the resultant image.

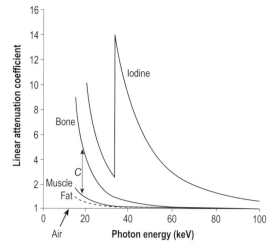

Fig. 3.21 The variation of linear attenuation coefficients as a function of photon energy for fat, muscle, bone and iodine.

- Reduced kV (see Fig. 3.21)
- Increased density (for Compton-dominant effects)
- Increased atomic number (for photoelectric-dominant effects)
- Presence of contrast media

Reduced contrast is caused by

- Scatter
- Higher kV

Magnification and distortion — Some important aspects of a radiological image arise simply from the fact that X-rays travel in straight lines. Fig. 3.22 shows how the image of a structure produced by a diverging X-ray beam is larger than the structure itself.

If the diagram were redrawn with larger or smaller values for F and h, it would be seen that magnification is reduced by using a longer focus-detector distance (F) or by decreasing the object-detector distance (h). When positioning the patient, the detector is therefore usually placed close to the structures of interest. If the tissues were compressed, this would also reduce patient dose. On the other hand, magnification may be helpful for visualising small detail, but this is generally used only in mammography.

$$Magnification = F/(F - h)$$

Distortion refers to a difference between the shape of an object and its appearance as an image. It may be caused by foreshortening of the shadow of a tilted object (e.g., a tilted circle appears as an ellipse). It may also be caused by differential magnification of the parts of a structure nearer

to or further away from the imaging device. It can be reduced by using a longer focus-detector distance.

Unsharpness and blurring: There are three types of unsharpness.

1. Geometric unsharpness/blurring: This contrasts with perfect sharpness, which represents an image of a stationary structure, produced from an ideal point source. Focal spots are not ideal point sources, but have a defined area (f, in Fig. 3.22). This causes a penumbra, which is the unsharpness/blurring at edges (P, in Fig. 3.22). Unsharpness can be expressed as:

$$U_g = fh/(F - h)$$

Geometric unsharpness (P) is reduced by:

- Decreasing focal spot size (f)
- Decreasing object-detector distance (h)
- Increasing focus-detector distance (F)

2. Movement unsharpness: The edge of a moving structure is difficult to discretely image. It is defined by:
   a. $U_m = vt$
      i. Where v = speed (m/s) and t = time (s)
   b. Movement unsharpness is reduced with:
      i. Immobilisation
      ii. Breath holding
      iii. Short exposure times

3. Absorption unsharpness: Rounded or tapered structures do not have well-defined edges. These appear with a gradated transition rather than a discrete edge (see Fig. 3.23).

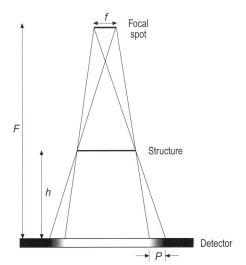

Fig. 3.22 Magnification of the X-ray image and geometrical unsharpness.

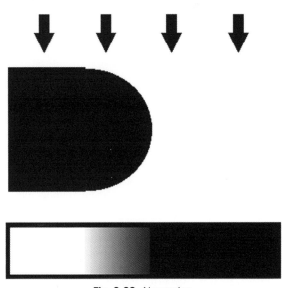

Fig. 3.23 Absorption.

Noise — Variation in levels of grey in an image, unrelated to the structure being imaged. This is also referred to as quantum mottle and is an inherent random variation in detected photons. It is determined by the number of photons *(N)*. The SNR is determined by $N/\sqrt{N}$; thus SNR is $\sqrt{N}$. To increase SNR, more X-rays *(N)* are required, through either an increase in flux (increased mA) or increased detector efficiency.

Resolution — This indicates the ability to distinguish between two objects (fine detail). In radiography, it represents the highest occurring frequency of lines that can be resolved in a high-contrast bar pattern. This is expressed in line pairs/mm and represents the MTF of the system. With the use of thin-film transistors, there is a limit to the number of line pairs possible compared with the detector element size. This is governed by the sampling pitch (the distance between the centres of adjacent detector elements). The sampling pitch determines the Nyquist frequency. Each pixel can record greyscale with a bit depth of 2^n values (where n is a bit; e.g., $2^9 = 512$ values of grey).

Contrast Media

Generally, there is low inherent contrast between soft tissues in the human body. To counter this, contrast agents are used to increase tissue differentiation. These agents need to have a high atomic number to maximise photoelectric absorption. Also, the absorption edge should be to the left of the spectrum exiting the patient. The most commonly used contrasts in radiographic imaging are:
- Iodine
  - Atomic number 53, $E_K = 33$ keV
- Barium
  - Atomic number 56, $E_K = 37$ keV
- Air
  - Very low density

Dual-Energy Radiography

This technique utilises the different responses of body tissues to low- and high-energy incident X-ray photons and can generate tissue-selective images. Calcium-containing tissues (e.g., bone) have a higher attenuation coefficient at lower keV (see Fig. 3.24).

There are two methods for dual-energy radiography:

Single exposure — Two storage phosphor plates are separated by a copper filter. The front plate receives unfractionated incident X-ray photons. The rear plate receives higher-energy photons (whereby the copper plate has filtered the lower keV). Weighted subtraction images from the two plates yield bone- and soft tissue —

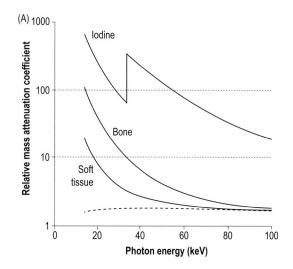

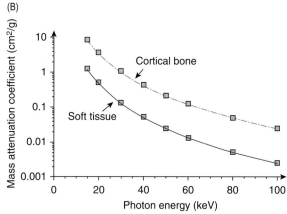

Fig. 3.24 Mass attenuation coefficients as a function of energy. Cortical bone vs soft tissue.

selective images. As there are fewer incident photons on the rear plate, there is a lower SNR in the tissue-selective image.

Dual exposure — Two sequential radiographs are obtained 200 ms apart. Two different energies are used, one at 60 kV and the other at 120 kV. There is a higher dose for this than the single-exposure method, but this yields an improved SNR. There is a small possibility of a misregistration artefact as there is a time interval between both exposures.

Regardless of method used, there are three images produced (see Fig. 3.25):
1. Standard unsubtracted image
2. Soft tissue-selective images
3. Bone-selective images

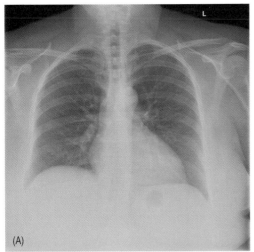

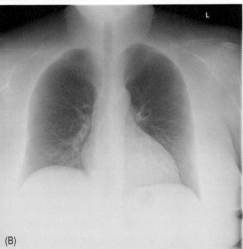

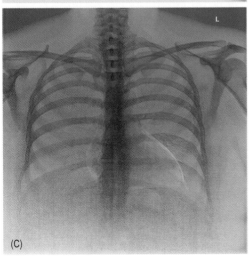

Fig. 3.25 Dual-energy chest X-ray. (A) Original image; (B) soft tissue-selective image; (C) bone-selective image.

MAMMOGRAPHY

Equipment

An overview of the equipment is shown in Figs. 3.26 and 3.27.

X-ray source on C-arm — Angled target orientation. The anode heel effect is utilised to align the higher-energy beam over the chest wall side. A beryllium exit window is used to minimise attenuation.

Compression paddle — The normal compression force deployed is 100—150 N. This helps to equalise breast tissue thickness. Compression also reduces the required radiation dose, scatter, and geometric and movement unsharpness.

For mammography, there is a fixed focus-detector distance of ~65 cm. A grid is not used in magnification views.

There are two sizes of fields of view: full and small.

Full-field size is the standard with craniocaudal (CC) or medial lateral oblique (MLO) views (see Fig. 3.28). These have a broad focal spot size of 0.3 mm.

The small field size is used for spot views. This view also requires focal compression using a small compression paddle (see Fig. 3.29), and has a focal spot size of 0.1—0.15 mm. This view allows for:

- Increased tissue separation
- Distinguish between true lesion and tissue overlap
- Increased resolution from decreased thickness

Automatic exposure control — This is integrated in the detector manifold. It functions based on limits determined before exposure. It can limit the exposure of higher-density breasts. It can be adjusted based on dose detected.

Stereo biopsy equipment — These are used to enable vacuum-assisted core biopsy (11-G to 14-G needle size with suction power of 23—25 mmHg). This equipment allows the three-dimensional (3D) localisation of a lesion, using either two additional views (±15°) or tomosynthesis. A special compression paddle with a central window is utilised. After biopsy, a radiopaque clip is left in the biopsy site. Secondary X-ray imaging of the biopsied samples is used to assess if microcalcifications are present (if part of target).

Target and Filter Materials

Mammography is different from other X-ray modalities. The main difference is that the breast has low inherent contrast. Breast tissue is a mixture of glandular and adipose which have similar radiographic characteristics. Breast imaging also requires very high spatial resolution to enable the detections of microcalcifications.

To enhance breast imaging, there are differences in the X-ray tube anode target and filters used. The target material should produce low-keV characteristic X-rays:

- 16—22 keV for normal breast size
- 20—30 keV for larger breasts

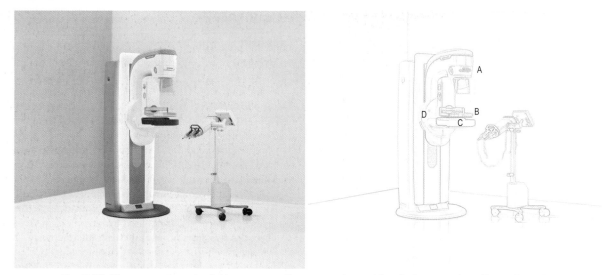

Fig. 3.26 Mammography unit. *A*, X-ray source; *B*, compression paddle; *C*, detector plate; *D*, rotating axle. (Credit Siemens Healthcare Ltd.)

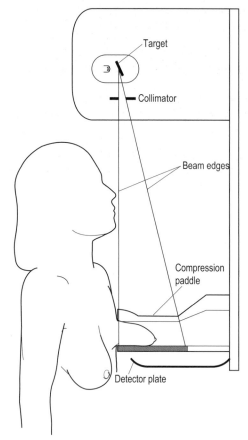

Fig. 3.27 Key components in a mammography unit.

The most common target is molybdenum (Mo), with characteristic X-rays at 17.4 keV and 19.6 keV. Rhodium (Rh) is also used with characteristic X-rays at 20.2 keV and 22.7 keV.

The filter is present to remove higher-energy X-ray photons, and trends towards monoenergetic beam production. Molybdenum has a K-edge of 20 keV. Rhodium has a K-edge of 23.3 keV.

Different target/filter combinations are used depending on the imaged breast. Molybdenum/molybdenum is most common (see Fig. 3.30). Molybdenum/rhodium or rhodium/rhodium combinations are used for larger patients or denser breasts (see Fig. 3.31).

A rhenium/molybdenum combination is not used as the molybdenum filter would attenuate the rhodium-characteristic X-rays.

Quality assurance — Optimisation of the mammography system is paramount due to it being a low-kV process. Any small changes in kV or processor conditions have a significantly larger effect than in other image modalities. Also, most mammograms are part of screening of healthy patients, and therefore doses should be minimised ('as low as reasonably practicable' principle). The quality assurance process for mammography is governed by IPEM (Institute of Physics and Engineering in Medicine, UK) 89.

Tomography and Tomosynthesis

Conventional projection radiography has 3 limitations, secondary to being a 2D representation of a 3D object.

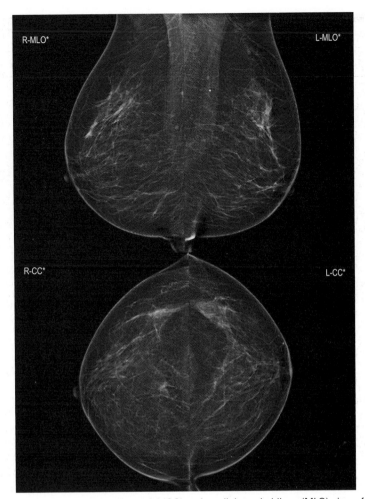

Fig. 3.28 Example of the standard craniocaudal (CC) and mediolateral oblique (MLO) views for right (R) and left (L).

These limitations include depth of individual components, the true shape of components, and the loss of contrast between similar density components.

Tomography attempts to overcome the loss of contrast between similar components and yield the true shape of components. Tomography consists of several imaged slices of the same object. Only structures in a selected slice (cut height) are imaged sharply. There is a higher overall radiation dose (~double).

In conventional mammography, there are two significant limitations:

- Sensitivity — In any single-plane image, dense tissue above or below the lesion of interest reduces visibility of the lesion
- Specificity — Two separate features that superimpose vertically (through plane) can appear as a lesion

Pseudotomographic imaging involves the acquisition of a limited number of projections to create a quasi-3D image of the breast. The process is governed by the angular range or sweep angle, which varies between manufacturers (15–50°). The number of projections acquired, scanning time, and tube motion (continuous vs

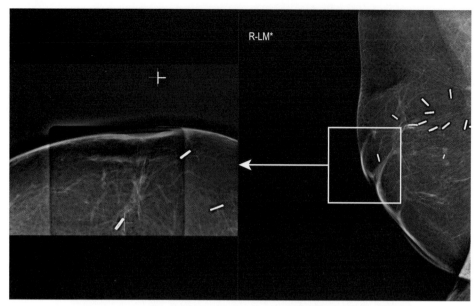

R-LM*

Fig. 3.29 Focal compression example.

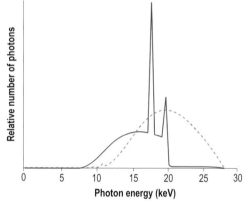

Fig. 3.30 The spectrum from a molybdenum target/filter (peaks at 17.4 keV and 19.6 keV), with the superimposed standard tungsten target/aluminium filter (dashed line).

step and shoot) are also manufacturer dependent. The detectors can be stationary or can rotate along with the X-ray tube. Angular range is defined by dose constraints (to minimise dose), with limited improvements in the incomplete Fourier imaging data. Figs. 3.32 and 3.33 outline the process of breast tomosynthesis and an example dataset acquired.

The X-Y resolution for tomosynthesis is comparable to full-field digital mammography (100–280 μm). There is increased Z-axis resolution which allows for depth separation (anisotropic voxels).

Further processing occurs with filtered back-projection, and iterative reconstruction algorithms used produce multiple slices parallel to the detector. This processing allows for improved detection of amorphous microcalcifications. Multiple slices can be summated into thick-slab images to better delineate microcalcifications.

Breast tomosynthesis is susceptible to specific artefacts:

- Blurring ripple — There is reduced volume averaging, leading to increased anatomic noise due to a small number of projections. High-density objects (including clips and markers) appear wider and less well defined with ripple artefacts (equal to the number of projections). The artefact is usually perpendicular to the X-ray tube sweep direction. It is less present in iterative reconstruction.

- Truncation — Some of the breast tissue is only covered by a few acquisitions but still contributes to the dataset:
  - 'Stair-step' effect (stepwise decrease in artefact presence)
  - 'Bright-edge' effect (overestimation of attenuation at the margins of the image)

- Loss of skin/superficial tissue — Large or dense breasts require higher radiation doses. X-rays which only travel through small tissue volumes, such as skin or superficial tissue, saturate the detector and lead to no signal detected from some parts of the imaged breast.

- Motion — The increased exposure times make patient movement more likely, which can be compounded if there is inadequate compression

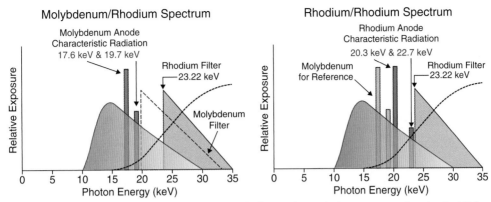

Fig. 3.31 Breast filter combinations. Dashed curve indicates the equivalent spectrum for standard X-Rays (Tungsten target / Aluminium filter).

FLUOROSCOPY

Whilst radiography relates to the recording of a single image produced by X-rays transmitted through the body, fluoroscopy relates to recording real-time images or image sequences. This has been traditionally facilitated by the image intensifier, available from the 1950s, and still in use in many centres at present. The flat panel detector has been available since 2000. On current fluoroscopy systems, any screen image can be saved as a spot image or screen grab. Fluorography refers to the acquisition of single diagnostic-quality images.

Equipment

Conventional equipment — This consists of a tube mounted under the bed, with the image intensifier above the table. The table position can vary (rotation or tilting). The operative controls are at the table (see Fig. 3.34). The position and angle of the tube or intensifier can also be changed.
Remote control equipment — Here, the tube is mounted over the bed, with the image intensifier underneath. The operative controls are remote to the table. There is high scattered dose, so a shielding screen is used to limit the operator dose. Fig. 3.35 demonstrates an example of the apparatus in an angiographic fluoroscopy suite.
C-arm — This can be fixed to a room, or portable for theatres (see Fig. 3.36)

Image Intensifier

The cross-section of an image intensifier is shown in Fig. 3.37.

Input screen — This is the quantum sink for the image intensifier. The window is composed of aluminium, titanium, or glass. There is low attenuation of incident X-rays. It is required to maintain the vacuum.

The phosphor is required to convert X-ray photons to light photons. It is composed of caesium iodide crystals with sodium (Fig. 3.38). These crystals are 0.3–0.45 mm thick and organised into a crystal lattice with high packing fraction. A needle structure is constructed to reduce lateral spread of light photons (similar to fibre-optics). The respective K-edges are at 36 keV for caesium and 33 keV for iodine. The phosphor absorbs 60% of incident X-rays. Each absorbed X-ray photon produces 1000–2000 light photons (blue spectrum).

The photocathode converts these produced light photons to electrons. The photocathode is composed of antimony caesium ($SbCs_3$). It is 20 nm thick and blue-light sensitive, but only 15% efficient. There are 200 electrons created per incident X-ray photon.

There is a 25-kV negative voltage compared to the anode at the output screen to facilitate electron movement towards the output screen. Additionally, the input screen is curved, based on the radius from the focal point of the electron beam to ensure the electrons travel the same distance to the output screen.

Electrostatic lens — This consists of 5 electrodes:
1. Photocathode
2. G1 — Resolution uniformity
3. G2 — Focus
4. G3 — Zoom
5. Anode
This lens allows for:
Magnification — The electron focus or crossover point is changed along the long axis. The output screen is

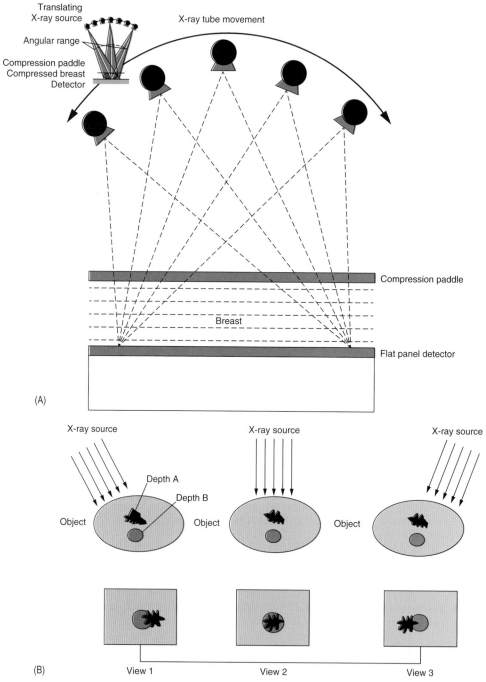

Fig. 3.32 Breast tomosynthesis. (A) Varying projections along an angular sweep about the breast with a stationary detector. (B) Paths of incident X-rays through the breast at different angles with resultant image on detector plate.

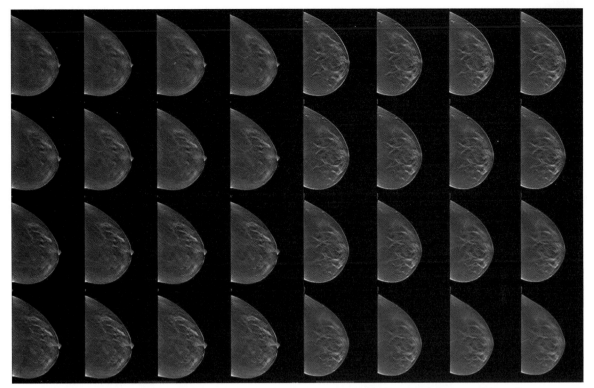

Fig. 3.33 Breast tomosynthesis example. All of these images are combined to form a quasi-three-dimensional image stack of the breast.

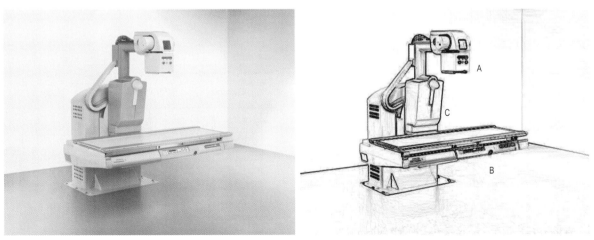

Fig. 3.34 Conventional fluoroscopy suite. *A,* X-ray tube; *B,* patient table with inbuilt controls, detector, can have foot stand attached to bottom; *C,* allows the table to rotate almost 90° to allow for standing examinations. (Credit Siemens Healthcare Ltd.)

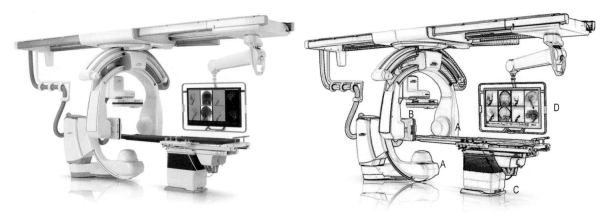

Fig. 3.35 Remote-controlled interventional radiography suite. *A*, X-ray sources (this example has two sources that can function like an ultrahigh pitch CT scanner to produce a three-dimensional reconstruction); *B*, detectors; *C*, patient table (often incorporates detachable controls that can be housed remotely); *D*, display screen. (Credit Siemens Healthcare Ltd.)

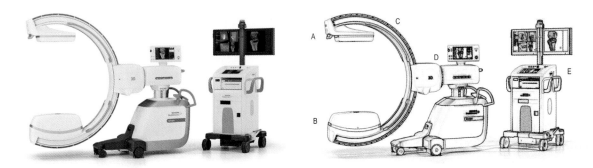

Fig. 3.36 C-arm. *A*, detector; *B*, X-ray source; *C*, C-arm allowing rotation about the Z-axis; *D*, rotation axle to allow change in the X-Y plane and cranial-caudal angulation; *E*, portable display and remote controls. (Credit Siemens Healthcare Ltd.)

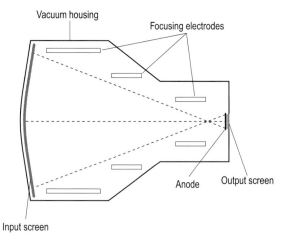

Fig. 3.37 Cross-section of an image intensifier.

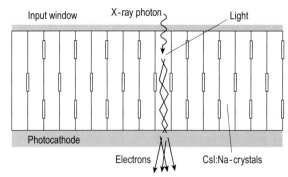

Fig. 3.38 Detailed view of the input screen of an image intensifier, demonstrating internal light reflection in the caesium iodide crystals.

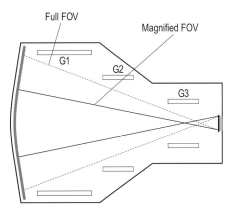

Fig. 3.39 Electron beam path in the image intensifier for a magnified field of view.

covered by the central input screen only (see Fig. 3.39). This helps to overcome limitations in the spatial resolution of the viewing screen. However, increased exposure is required to maintain brightness, and some brightness is lost as there is reduced minification gain.
Minification — This reflects intensification caused by reducing image size from input to output screen, governed by:

$$(\text{input screen/output screen})^2$$

Flux gain — Each electron from the photocathode produces numerous light photons at the output phosphor (~ 50) due to increased energy from acceleration through voltage potential across the system

$$\text{Brightness gain} = \text{Minification gain} \times \text{flux gain}$$

Output screen — Here, the electrons are converted to light. The material used is zinc cadmium sulphide doped with silver (ZnCdS:Ag). This is usually 4—8 μm thick (it does not need to be thicker as there is limited range of incident electrons, and this also ensures very little light spread in the layer). Additionally, there is a thin layer of aluminium to prevent backscatter of light photons (which would interact with the input screen and cause a cascade).

Optical Output

This component transmits light from the output phosphor of the image intensifier. There is feedback to the X-ray generator to ensure adequate output intensity. TV cameras are no longer used and have been replaced with CCDs and active-pixel sensors. The output viewing matrix is 512 × 512 with 8-bit greyscale. Temporal resolution is prioritised over spatial resolution.

Charge Coupled Devices (CCDs)

CCDs are widely incorporated into modern technologies and consist of a solid-state device of pixel detectors. They are fast and sensitive, with minimal burn-in and excellent thermal, electrical, and magnetic stability.

Pixel detectors have image capture and frame storage regions. Each detector contains semiconductor capacitors with photosensitive elements named detector elements (DELs). An incident light photon creates an electron-hole pair. These released electrons accumulate in a potential well. This yields a charge indicative of incident radiation dose. Image capture regions work by integrating the charge from the photosensitive elements over a set period, which is governed by the frame rate (usually 25 Hz). The charge is then transferred to the frame store region (pixel clocking). This charge is measured as a voltage which is digitised to greyscale to form the output image. The frame storage information is read to form an image whilst image capture concurrently acquires a new image.

There are 3 possible modes of acquisition (see Fig. 3.40):
1. Full frame — The entire image area is active. This is a slower process that requires mechanical shuttering during read-out.
2. Frame transfer — In this mode, half of the light-sensitive silicon area is shielded. The image is transferred from an active to shielded area for read-out. This requires twice the area of silicon.
3. Interline transfer — Every other line is shielded. This is a much faster process but half as efficient.

Active-Pixel Sensor

These have recently superseded CCD sensors. Each pixel sensor unit cell (dexel) has a photodetector and transistor. These are less expensive and simpler to construct than CCDs. There is better control of blooming, with less power consumption. Image processing is included in the in same circuit. These devices do suffer from increased noise and the rolling shutter effect.

Flat Panel Detector

These have replaced the traditional image intensifier system. They are similar to indirect detectors used in DR. These do not require a TV camera to convert output window signal to electronic signal. There are several advantages, including:

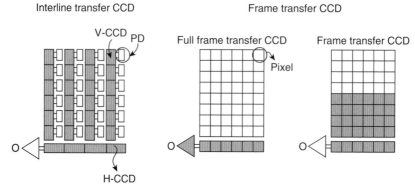

Fig. 3.40 CCD acquisition modes. *V-CCD,* Vertical CCD; *H-CCD,* horizontal CCD; *O,* output.

1. Reduced artefact:
   a. No geometrical distortion
   b. No vignetting
   c. Uniform response across field of view
   d. Digital process in entirety (no electronic noise)
2. Superior ergonomics facilitated by smaller components
3. Improved DQE
4. Extended dynamic range: 5000:1 vs 500:1 for II/TV system
5. Same spatial resolution for all fields of view:
   a. Determined by distance between centre of two adjacent detector elements (pitch):
      i. Max spatial resolution = $1/(2 \times pitch)$
      ii. Typically 2.5–3.2 lp/mm
   b. Fill factor = (sensitive area of detector element)/ $(pitch^2)$
      i. See Fig. 3.14
   c. Normally 60%–80% (read-out electronics are a finite size)
6. Reduced dose: The spatial resolution is the same for all fields of view. The X-ray flux is the same upon each detector element. There is a small increase in dose applied to reduce noise at a rate of 1/field-of-view when the field of view is decreased.
7. Data storage
   a. Quantisation – allocation of input signal into a certain bin, based on number of bins available. Governed by bit depth (2^n discrete levels [n number of bits]). As the number of bits/bins increases, so does the accuracy of the recorded input signal.
   b. Significant increase in data size allocated to digital fluoroscopy

Automatic Brightness Control

This is an important mechanism to ensure constant brightness of fluoroscopy images. It is also referred to as an automatic exposure control system in fluorography. This control system requires electronic sampling of output display signal, or output phosphor of the image intensifier. From this, there are automatic adjustments of the kV or mA (see Fig. 3.41). The adjustments are governed by 'patient dose rate' mode (see Fig. 3.42):

- Curve A – anti-isowatt curve. Increase in mA and kV as radiological thickness increases. There are pre-set maximum mA/kV values, with 400 W maximum.
- Curve B – iodine contrast imaging. Holds kV at 60–65 kV, the optimum spectrum for imaging iodine. Only the mA is increased up to ~6.5 mA (400 W/62 kV = 6.5 mA). This curve has high image quality but high dose.
- Curve C – high-kV curve. This is a dose-minimisation curve, used mostly in paediatrics.

Dose Rates

Dose depends on several factors. These include screening time, DQE of the image intensifier, and the acceptable noise for study type (level of detail required at each image). Screening time varies based on indication, with orthopaedic at a few seconds, barium contrast at a few minutes, and angiography at 15 min or more.

Pulsed fluoroscopy is used to reduce dose rate in angiographic imaging. In this process, the X-ray generator is switched on and off to supply pulses of X-rays, where 'continuous' is equivalent to 25–30 pulses/s (each individual pulse lasts 2–20 ms). The rate can be reduced to 15, 7.5,

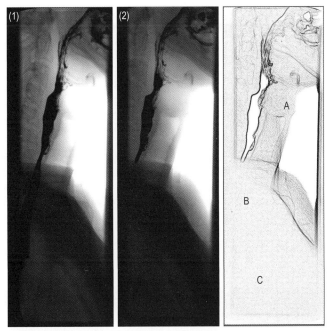

Fig. 3.41 Automatic brightness control in a barium swallow examination, with two different settings (1 and 2). In image (1), region A is not discernible, with the attempts of the machine to make region C visible. At region B, there is limited image quality due to the amount of body traversed by the X-ray photons.

or 3.75 pulses/s, etc. Despite the rapid switching, there is no flickering as each image is retained until a new image is generated, and the critical flicker frequency is not exceeded.

Digital Fluorography

Some images acquired are at higher doses than for fluoroscopy. These are usually digital spot images of diagnostic quality (see Fig. 3.43). The acquisition matrix is 1024 × 1024, with a 10-bit greyscale. These images are of high mA, but reduced quantum mottle. The dose equivalent is for 2 s or 0.1–5 μGy.

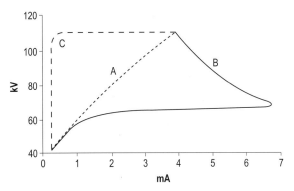

Fig. 3.42 Relationship between kilovoltage (kV) and milliamperage (mA) used for automatic brightness control. Curve A is an anti-isowatt curve, curve B is optimised for iodine contrast imaging, and curve C is for low-dose high-kV fluoroscopy.

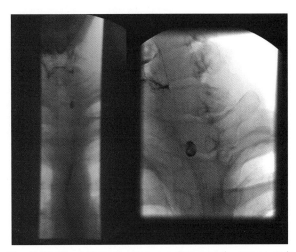

Fig. 3.43 The left image shows a fluoroscopic screen grab taken during a fluoroscopic run. The right image shows the increased resolution available with fluorography settings.

Digital Subtraction Angiography

This technique produces images of contrast-filled vessels, isolated from other tissues. The steps to enable this are as follows:

1. Non-contrast image acquired

This acquired image undergoes processing with histogram normalisation and is then stored as a mask (see Fig. 3.44A). Multiple masks can be stored based on table position.

2. Contrast image(s) acquired

Contrast is injected and new images are acquired. The non-contrast image mask is subtracted pixel by pixel from the contrast image, yielding a subtraction image. This subtraction allows for higher clarity of contrast-filled vessels (see Fig. 3.44B). The subtraction images can be either single images, or 'runs.'

Temporal averaging is a process that increase signal for static objects. It is achieved through recursive software filtering, whereby values from previous acquired images are added to the current image. This process yields less noise as noise is a random process. Whilst it can improve signal for static objects, there is loss of signal for moving objects.

Digital subtraction angiography is prone to artefacts just like other techniques:

1. Movement — This causes misregistration between the mask and contrast images. It is possible to compensate with pixel shifting by the processing software. Failing this, a new mask should be acquired.

2. High-contrast interface boundaries — This can lead to loss of image detail at these interfaces.

3. Bowel gas movement — This affects the accuracy of the mask and can lead to persistent bowel gas artefact on the contrast images (see Fig. 3.45; Boxes 3.1 and 3.2).

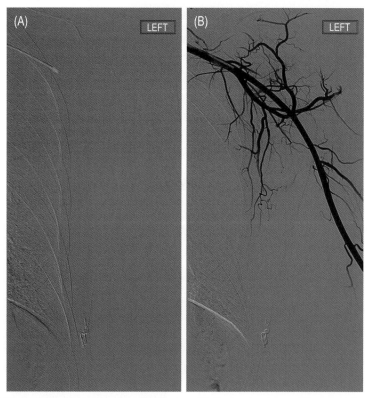

Fig. 3.44 (A) Mask of the region of a left axillary artery. (B) Contrast-enhanced fluoroscopic run after mask applied.

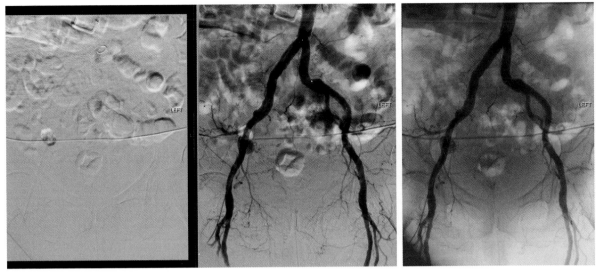

Fig. 3.45 Persistence of bowel gas on a mask image and subsequent fluoroscopic runs.

BOX 3.1   Dose in Fluoroscopy

Minimising Patient Dose
- Tight collimation of X-ray beam
- Increased filtration
- Increase source-skin distance
- Limit distance between patient and II/FPD entrance
- Remove anti-scatter grid, especially in children
- Dose spreading: rotation of system to prevent persistent imaging over one section of skin only
- Pulsed fluoroscopy rather than continuous, best at lower frame-rate acquisition
- Use of magnification only when necessary
- Last-image-hold: previously acquired image is displayed on screen for evaluation
- Electronic collimation: overlay of a collimator on last image to adjust field of view

Dose to Staff Is Mostly From Stray Radiation
- Scatter is the biggest contribution to staff dose

Minimising Staff Dose
- Personal shielding: lead apron, leaded glasses, thyroid collars
- Mobile shielding: leaded table drapes, ceiling-/table-suspended shielding screens
- Maintain maximum possible distance from patient
- Individual staff dose monitoring
- Optimisation of technique dose
  - Collimation
  - Exposure time
  - Exposure rate

BOX 3.2   Quality Assurance

Requirement of IRR 1999
  Incorporates a framework to oversee:
Commissioning of new equipment
Performance tests
Patient dose assessment
  Involves radiation protection adviser
  Most medical equipment quality assurance is based on
IPEM Report 91
Physical parameter to be tested
Frequency
Priority
  Level 1 good practice
  Level 2 best practice, but not essential
Level of expertise required to perform process

Level A
Radiographer performed; frequently performed; relatively quick and simple;
Level B
Greater expertise required (usually medical physicist); more rarely performed; can require complex equipment with detailed analysis of results
Action levels
Remedial
  Action is required on the equipment, but it can be used in the interim
Suspension
  Immediate removal of equipment from clinical use

FURTHER READING

Balter S. Fluoroscopic frame rates: not only dose. *AJR Am J Roentgenol.* 2014;203:W234–W236.

Beckett KR, Moriarity AK, Langer JM. Safe use of contrast media: what the radiologist needs to know. *Radiographics.* 2015;35:1738–1750.

Bor D, others. Investigation of grid performance using simple image quality tests. *J Med Phys.* 2015;41:21–28.

Curry TS, Dowdey JE, Murry RE. *Christensen's Physics of Diagnostic Radiology.* 4th ed. Philadelphia: Lea & Febiger; 1990.

Heidbuchel H, others. Practical ways to reduce radiation dose for patients and staff during device implantations and electrophysiological procedures. *Europace.* 2014;16:946–964.

Hernanz-Schulman M, others. Pause and pulse: ten steps that help manage radiation dose during pediatric fluoroscopy. *AJR Am J Roentgenol.* 2011;197:475–481.

Huda W, Abrahams RB. Radiographic techniques, contrast, and noise in x-ray imaging. *AJR Am J Roentgenol.* 2015;204: W126–W131.

Kuhlman JE, others. Dual-energy subtraction chest radiography: what to look for beyond calcified nodules. *Radiographics.* 2006;26:79–92.

Mall S, others. The role of digital breast tomosynthesis in the breast assessment clinic: a review. *J Med Imaging Radiat Sci.* 2017;64:203–211.

Meisinger QC, others. Radiation protection for the fluoroscopy operator and staff. *AJR Am J Roentgenol.* 2016;207:745–754.

Nickoloff EL. AAPM/RSNA physics tutorial for residents: physics of flat-panel fluoroscopy systems: survey of modern fluoroscopy imaging: flat-panel detectors versus image intensifiers and more. *Radiographics.* 2011;31:591–602.

Seibert JA. Flat-panel detectors: how much better are they? *Pediatr Radiol.* 2006;36:173–181.

Shetty CM, others. Computed radiography image artifacts revisited. *AJR Am J Roentgenol.* 2011;196:W37–W47.

Tirada N, others. Digital breast tomosynthesis: physics, artifacts, and quality control considerations. *Radiographics.* 2019;39:413–426.

Walz-Flannigan AI, others. Pictorial review of digital radiography artifacts. *Radiographics.* 2018;38:833–846.

Computed Tomography

Computed tomography (CT) was introduced in the early 1970s. It was originally termed 'computed axial tomography' (CAT), to emphasise the key role of the computer, and to distinguish it from conventional tomography techniques. Methods of image reconstruction that could be used for CT had been formulated many decades before its introduction but only as a branch of abstract mathematics. It was with the advent of the digital computer that theory could become practice, and it is in large part because of the developments in computer technology over the succeeding years that the technique has been transformed from basic transaxial imaging to true 3D (and 4D with multiphase imaging) representations of the body.

The CT scan is now a mainstay of the radiology department, with busy departments having multiple machines.

BASICS OF THE CT SCANNER

The basic overview of a modern CT scanner is shown in Figs. 4.1 and 4.2. It is housed in a lead-lined room, to prevent irradiation of adjacent rooms and corridors. There are 3 main parts:

Patient table — This is where the patient is located for the duration of the scan. The patient table traverses through the gantry perpendicular to the aperture (along the Z-axis). The table moves in and out of the scanner during preparation and acquisition of images (machine or operator dependent). It has some degree of movement allowing for elevation and descent compared to the floor. Each patient table has varying weight limits.

Gantry — This houses the main hardware of the CT scanner. It contains the X-ray tube, the collimator, filter, and detectors, all mounted within a slip ring. The slip ring is a fundamental component of the modern CT scanner. It facilitates continuous rotation and maintains electrical power and detector signal transmission. It uses a system of brushes and rings to facilitate sliding contact, with newer systems using optical data channels for detector output. The gantry also has a small control panel for some manual operation, if required. The gantry is connected by multiple transmission cables to the control room.

Control room — This is where the operation of the CT scanner is controlled. The computer in this room allows interface for electronic selection of patient, selection of CT study, storage of acquired raw data, and reconstruction of CT images for picture archival and communication systems (PACS). Other control systems may be present, such as the pump control for intravenous contrast injection (also see Box 4.1).

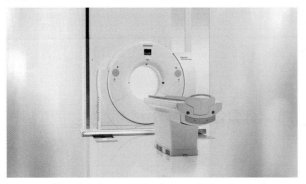
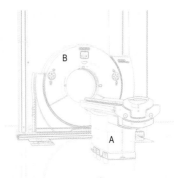

Fig. 4.1 An example of a standard computed tomography scanner. *A*, patient table; *B*, gantry. Not shown: Operator console and computer units. (Credit: Siemens Healthcare Ltd.)

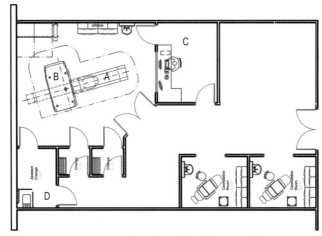

Fig. 4.2 Computed tomography room layout. *A*, patient table; *B*, gantry; *C*, operator control room; *D*, patient changing rooms. (Credit: Siemens Healthcare Ltd.)

CT COMPONENTS USED IN IMAGE ACQUISITION

X-ray tube — Similar to that used in conventional radiography an X-ray tube for CT scanning operates between 80 and 140 kV. The tube current operates at up to 1000 mA, which undergoes modulation during scanning based on the patient's topogram. The X-ray tube will often have two focal spot sizes. X-ray tubes in CT have high heat capacity as CT has longer scan times than conventional radiography, and heat capacity can exceed 4 MJ. As in conventional radiography, ~99% of the energy produced in the X-ray tube is converted to heat. Anode heat dissipation is ~10 kW. The Straton tube was developed in the

early 2000s by Siemens and allows conductive heat loss from the anode rather than the usual radiation in a vacuum.

Collimator — This is mounted on the X-ray tube to reduce scatter and irradiation of patient. The variable aperture sizes control the Z-axis beam width (size).

Filter — There are two methods for filtration of the X-ray beam.

1. Bow-tie filter — The noise levels are poorly matched over the X-Y/transaxial plane of the patient. The lowest dose and highest noise occurs in the centre of the patient, whilst the highest dose occurs at the peripheries. A bow-tie filter is used to equalise transmitted intensities across the patient (see Fig. 4.4B).

BOX 4.1 Scanner Generations

The earliest clinical computed tomography scanner had an X-ray source and a single detector (Fig. 4.3A). Data acquisition involved moving both tube and detector across the scanning plane to acquire a series of transmission measurements. The detector and tube were then rotated by 1° and the process repeated. In all, data was collected through a 180° rotation. This scanner may be referred to as the *rotate–translate* type. To reduce scan times, the next generation of scanner had, instead of a single detector, a bank of up to 30 detectors that could measure data simultaneously but that were still insufficient to cover the full cross-section of the patient (Fig. 4.3B). Therefore, the rotate–translate procedure was still needed, but it became possible to reduce scan times from just under 5 min for the earliest scanner to less than 20 s. Note that these are the data acquisition times for a single slice. Inevitably, these two early designs became known as *first* and *second generation*.

The logical next step in scanner technology was of the type described in this chapter; that is, a scanner with a large number of small detectors arranged in an arc to cover the complete cross-section of the patient. This eliminated the requirement for the linear translation of tube and detectors and allowed for continuous data collection through a full 360° rotation. This may be described as a *rotate–rotate* or *third-generation scanner* (Fig. 4.3C).

One of the technological problems with early scanners was detector stability, and this was made worse by the movement of the gantry. This and other problems led to the development of a *fourth-generation* or *rotate–stationary scanner*, in which the detectors were arranged in a stationary ring outside the path of the rotating tube (Fig. 4.3D). This overcame some of the problems of detector stability and made reconstruction simpler. An additional advantage was that the outer part of the fan beam would always pass outside the patient, and during each rotation every detector would be able to measure unattenuated radiation. This measurement could be used to adjust the calibration of each detector throughout the scanning cycle. However, the downside to the design is that the total number of detectors is increased by a factor of about 6, and this becomes prohibitive, particularly with multi-slice scanners. In addition, higher doses are required because of the increased distance between the patient and the detectors since the tube has to rotate within the detector ring.

A so-called *fifth-generation scanner*, more correctly referred to as an electron-beam scanner, was introduced in the early 1980s. It employed an electron source that produced an electron beam that could be focused on to and swept round a high-voltage target ring that covered a 210° arc below the patient. X-rays would be produced and following collimation detected above the patient on an offset 216° ring of detectors. There were no mechanical parts, so the electron beam could be swept across the full arc in no more than 50 ms. This rapid imaging time permitted imaging of the heart, for which the system was originally designed.

The *generation* terminology for describing scanners is now obsolete. With the advent of multi-slice scanners, the rotate–rotate geometry of the third-generation scanner has become an industry standard. These scanners now have up to 320 detector rows, can achieve temporal resolution of 75 ms, achieve a spatial resolution of 0.28 mm, and utilise dual-source scanners and hybrid reconstruction algorithms.

2. Inherent window filtration is 6 mm aluminium (copper has been used previously). This removes low-energy X-rays that only contribute to dose. This reduces beam hardening.

Detectors

Requirements — Detectors need to be small (≤ 1 mm), with a very small dead space (inter-detector separation). They need high detection efficiency and a fast response with negligible afterglow. They also need to have a wide dynamic operating range and be stable.

Solid-state detector — This consists of a scintillator and photodiode all within 0.5 mm^2 (area) × 1 mm (depth). The scintillator (cadmium tungstate, bismuth germinate, rare earth ceramic) converts the incident X-ray to a light photon. The photodiode converts light photons to an electrical signal. Overall, there is high detection efficiency ($\sim 90\%$) and high geometrical efficiency ($\sim 80\%$), with negligible afterglow.

Multiple Rows of Detectors

This arrangement helps facilitate isotropic voxel achievement. Each row has around 800 detectors (in the transaxial or X-Y plane). Faster scan times are achievable as multiple slices acquired at once. Most detector sizes are limited to 0.5 mm^2 or 0.625 mm^2. Spatial resolution of up to 0.28 mm is currently marketed as achievable. A 128-slice scanner has 128 detectors along the Z-axis (some manufacturers currently claim 640 slices with 320 detectors along the Z-axis).

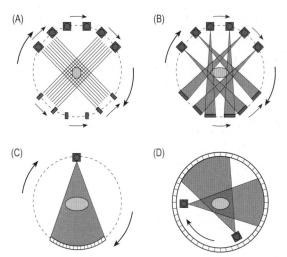

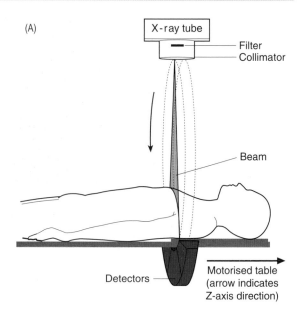

Fig. 4.3 Illustration of the development of the computed to-mography scanner from (A) first to (D) fourth generation.

Array types — There are 3 types of arrays (see Fig. 4.5).
1. Linear array — every detector is the same size
2. Adaptive array — thinner central detector sizes, which get progressively wider to away from centre
3. Hybrid array — narrow central detectors, larger outside detectors

OPERATION OF A CT SCANNER

After the patient is placed in the CT table, several steps occur in the acquisition of a CT scan. The initial step involves determining patient orientation: prone/supine/lateral and head-feet orientation. This step is vital as the acquired datasets will have embedded anterior, posterior, right, and left markers based on this determined orientation.

The next step is the scanned projection radiograph (also called scout image or topogram). To acquire this image, the patient table moves along the Z-axis for a distance defined by the operator. The X-ray tube is pre-set to either the 12 o'clock position for a frontal topogram or 3/9 o'clock for the lateral topogram. The X-ray tube does not rotate during this acquisition, with collimation set to the narrowest slice width. Multiple 2D slices through the patient are acquired as the patient moves through the gantry. These are summed to form a topogram (similar to a radiograph, see Fig. 4.6). This topogram is then used to plan the CT volume acquisition, particularly for dose modulation and total anatomical region of interest. After regions of interest are set, steps such as breathing instructions, contrast timings, and multiphase CT acquisition are set.

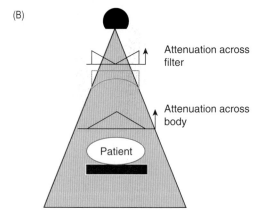

Fig. 4.4 (A) Components of a CT scanner withing the gantry; (B) Representation of the projection of the X-ray beam across the transaxial plane of the patient, with attenuation profile caused by the filter.

After the raw data from the CT scan has been acquired, this is reconstructed into the images stored on PACS.

IMAGE ACQUISITION

Helical and Multi-slice Scanners

Helical scanning — This is also known as volume or spiral acquisition. It involves the continuous rotation of the gantry (enabled with slip-ring technology). There is continuous acquisition of data as the gantry table moves

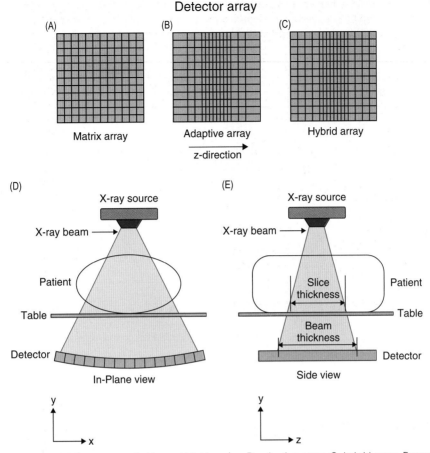

Fig. 4.5 Array types. Array types: A, Linear / Matrix array; B, adaptive array; C, hybrid array. Perpendicular views of the X-ray beam during image acquisition with in-plane (D) and side (E) views, demonstrating relative slice and beam thicknesses. The detector is constructed of one of the array types A–C.

along the Z-axis (table feed, see Fig. 4.7). In this process, no single transaxial slice is irradiated – all 'slices' are interpolated. To enable interpolation for image recon-struction, a full 180° plus fan angle (usually 30–60°) is required. The slice thickness is determined by collimator length and is limited by detector-row width.

$$Pitch = \frac{Tabletop\ movement\ per\ rotation\ (also\ called\ table\ feed)}{slice\ thickness\ (collimator\ length)}$$

where a pitch of 1 means no overlap or separation of the acquired data, >1 implies a gap in data acquisition, and <1 implies overlap in data acquisition.

Data interpolation: See Fig. 4.8. The data at Z^*XY^* is interpolated given the values at Z_1XY_1 and Z_2XY_2, with weighting based on distance to Z_1XY_1 (D_1). Slice width

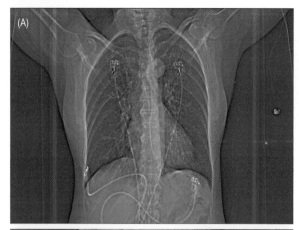

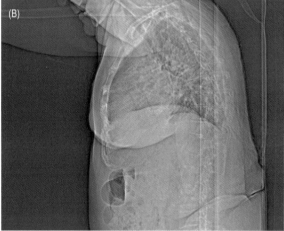

Fig. 4.6 Scout image or topogram. *A*, AP view; *B*, lateral view.

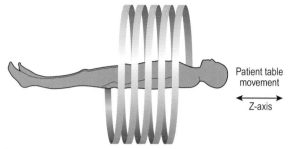

Fig. 4.7 The change in position of the collimated beam for a single-slice helical scanner.

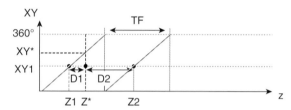

Fig. 4.8 Slice interpolation. The position of the beam through the patient is represented by purple lines. These are separated by the distance corresponding to the table feed *(TF)*.

minimum is limited to the size of the individual detector elements.

Advantages of helical scanning:
1. Minimises slice misregistration secondary to breathing
   – Scan can be acquired in one breath hold
2. Can acquire multiple contrast phases
   – Pre-contrast, arterial, venous, delayed
3. Pitch >1 reduces exposure time and dose
   – Most above 1.5 are not clinically appropriate

Multi-slice scanner – Further evolution of the helical scanner to use detector arrays (see Fig. 4.5). These arrays enable multiple slices to be acquired simultaneously. Acquired slice thickness in multi-slice acquisition is determined by a few factors: (1) individual detector width (minimum slice thickness possible), (2) row width (maximum slice thickness possible), and (3) beam width (determined by degree of collimation)

Multi-slice pitch – Table feed/Thickness of acquired slices acquired simultaneously

IMAGE RECONSTRUCTION

The raw data acquired is a huge dataset in terms of information. As such, the raw data is not stored for use and is reconstructed through several techniques into more readily transferrable and usable datasets. There are 3 main reconstruction methods: back projection, filtered back projection, and iterative reconstruction. Whilst current standard CT scanners acquire raw data at an equivalent voxel size of 0.625 mm, the reconstruction techniques produce image datasets at voxel sizes of 1, 2, and 5 mm; 1 mm is used for lung and 2 mm is common for soft tissue.

Back projection – An algorithm that uses multiple single-point measurements about an axis of rotation of the object ('pencil beam' – line integral of the attenuation coefficient along the path) (Figs. 4.9 and 4.10). These are summed to form an image. This is not a sharp image – it often yields a star-artefact pattern from high-density objects. The algorithm is based on the following assumptions to create an 'ideal' system: the X-ray focal spot is a point source, the distribution of photons is considered uniform (ignores statistical distribution and noise), each detector is considered uniform in shape and size, and the cone-beam

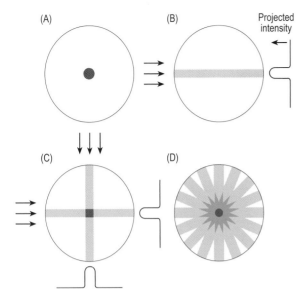

Fig. 4.9 The back-projection reconstruction technique. (A) A cylindrical body with a hole running through its centre; (B) the back-projected image for a single beam; (C) the image combined with a second orthogonal beam; and (D) the reconstructed image for eight beams.

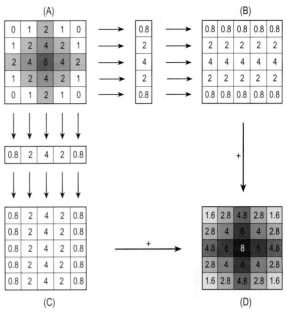

Fig. 4.10 Reconstruction of a 5 × 5 matrix of values using back projection. In this case, the object is represented by a 5 × 5 matrix with cell values as shown (A). Two projections are considered. The summed values are 'projected' back as the average value of the five cells in each row and column (B) and (C), and the two back-projected images are then summed to give the final representation shown in (D). The final representation is an approximate representation of the relative values.

shape of the X-ray beam is considered as a pencil beam instead.

Filtered back projection (FBP) — A convolution method. The logarithmic data of the projection profile is obtained. Each of these datasets are convolved with a digital filter (kernel — see below) and subsequently back-projected. Neighbouring data beams interact depending on distance from each other (summation). This process reduces blurring but is affected by noise and streak artefacts. This method can produce images with reconstruction angles of 180° rather than 360°.

Iterative reconstruction — This technique has recently re-entered the CT reconstruction arsenal. Previously, this technique was prohibited by time, but increased computing power has mitigated this. Some use an initial FBP image to start the iterative process (hybrid reconstruction). The difference between the generated image and the expected image is then used to further produce further iterations. Multiple iterations are processed to approximate the generated image closer to the expected image (see Fig. 4.11 for a graphical overview of the process). The overall process is limited by pre-determined cut-offs. In iterative reconstruction, there is reduced image noise and reduced dose. The techniques are mostly vendor-specific algorithms.

Reconstruction kernels and the raw data: There are multiple reconstruction kernels used in the convolution process of FBP and iterative reconstruction. These have predefined functions (e.g., edge detection, blurring, sharpening), and are specific to each machine. There are different kernels for lung, soft tissue, bone, and brain, among others. The raw data itself remains only on the scanner and is not transferred to PACS as it is a very large dataset. It is therefore paramount that any desired reconstruction is performed at time of acquisition, otherwise it will not be possible after the raw data has been deleted (on busy scanners, the raw data is often deleted weekly). An example of this is a case where only lung kernel reconstructions of a chest CT were sent to PACS, but not the soft tissue reconstructions. As both use a different kernel, it is not possible to replicate a true soft tissue dataset using the lung reconstruction. Differences in the kernel are shown in Fig. 4.12.

CT numbers — attenuation coefficient for each pixel is converted into a number

$$\text{CT number} = K\,(\mu - \mu_{\text{water}})/(\mu_{\text{water}})$$

where $K = 1000$ (CT numbers are Hounsfield units);
μ = attenuation coefficient

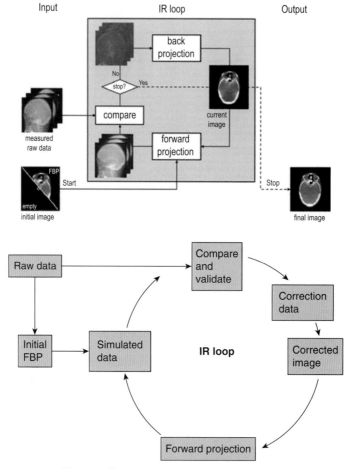

Fig. 4.11 Flow chart for iterative reconstruction.

IMAGE QUALITY

Resolution indicates the ability to distinguish between two objects. In CT imaging, it is often defined in line pairs per centimetre (usually 10–16 lp/cm). The resolution of the CT imaging system is defined by the modulation transfer function (MTF). This plots the spatial frequency vs image fidelity. For the ideal system, this plot should be flat (unity response — the system responds perfectly at all frequencies). The true curve is shown in Fig. 4.13. The fall-off in fidelity as the frequency increases allows for a comparison between different CT imaging systems. The MTF is often quoted at values of interest: 50%, 10%, and 0%. The system spatial resolution is influenced by several factors:

1. Focal spot size and shape:
- Small spot size ~0.4–0.7 mm: this has a higher resolution, but has a limited maximum mA (due to heat production)
- Large spot size ~1.0–1.2 mm: lower resolution

2. Detector cell size
- Smaller detectors yield higher spatial resolution
- Dead space between detectors contributes to loss of spatial resolution and must be minimised

3. Field of view — This refers to the transaxial area that is to be reconstructed. It relates to pixel and matrix size with the following equation:

$$\text{Pixel size} = \frac{\text{field of view}}{\text{matrix size}}$$

- The matrix size is often 512 × 512 (in X-Y plane). For example, if the field of view is 350 mm (× 350 mm), and the matrix is 512 (× 512), the pixel size is 0.7 mm (voxel XY size is 0.7 mm). A varying number of detectors contribute to each pixel/voxel depending on the chosen field of view (given that matrix size is fixed).

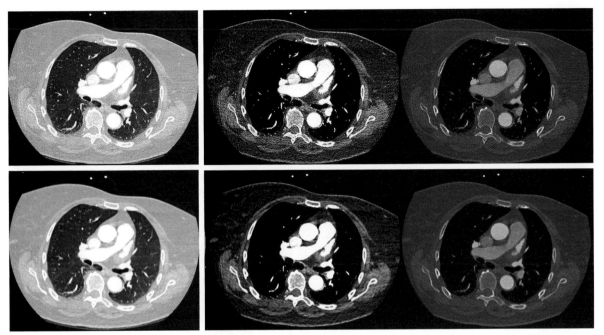

Fig. 4.12 Reconstruction kernels. Top row: Lung reconstruction kernel (increased edge detection, but noisier image) at lung, soft tissue, and bone windows. Bottom row: Soft tissue reconstruction kernel at lung, soft tissue, and bone windows. Despite the same histogram processing, the matched images are different.

TABLE 4.1 Approximate Range of CT Numbers for Various Tissues	
Tissue	**Range of CT Numbers**
Bone	>1000
Muscle	40–60
Liver	40–50
Brain (grey matter)	35–45
Brain (white matter)	20–30
Air	−1000
Fat	−50 to −100
Lung	−300 to −800

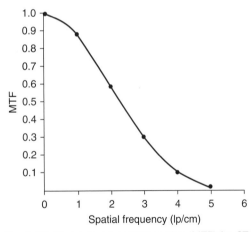

Fig. 4.13 Modulation transfer function (MTF) for CT.

- Pixel size is affected by the Nyquist theory, which states that the sampling frequency needs to be at least twice the highest frequency in the signal.

$$\text{Highest spatial frequency} = \text{Pixel size} / 2$$

4. Reconstruction algorithm
- Kernel can increase softness or sharpness

5. Additional factors affect the cross-plane resolution (Z-plane). The aim is to achieve an isotropic dataset. An isotropic voxel is a cube (X/Y/Z-axis dimensions are the same size). This enables 3D reconstruction and image manipulation (see Fig. 4.14). The Z-axis voxel dimension is governed by slice width and

detector length along the Z-axis. There is also overlap of acquired data in the Z-axis depending on pitch.

- Temporal resolution — There is an inherent time required for an image to be acquired. In this time, the patient can directly (e.g., breathing out) or indirectly (e.g., heartbeat) move. Temporal resolution refers to the ability of a scanner to take a 'still image.' This is predominantly important in cardiac imaging. Two of the main methods to reduce the time required for image acquisition are:
1. Half-scan — 180° rotation plus fan angle (220° total), rather than a full rotation. This requires a specific half-scan algorithm to reconstruct.

2. Dual-source imaging — The CT scanner gantry contains two X-ray sources, mounted at 90° to each other. With one-quarter rotation, these dual sources cause a half scan to be detected.

Noise

Noise affects all electronic systems. For CT imaging, it reduces the quality of the produced image. Noise will decrease the contrast resolution of small objects and the spatial resolution of low-contrast objects. There are three types of noise:

- Quantum noise — This is caused by a lack of sufficient photons. The average X-ray flux (called M) for each

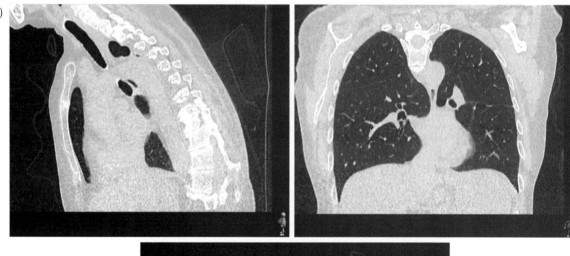

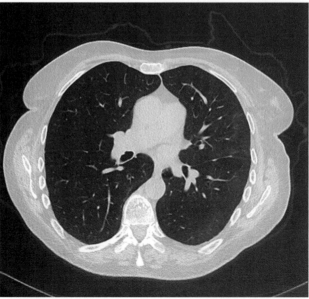

Fig. 4.14 (A) Isotropic voxel dataset. The X/Y/Z axis dimensions are equal yielding images that appear of the same resolution in all 3 planes.

(B)

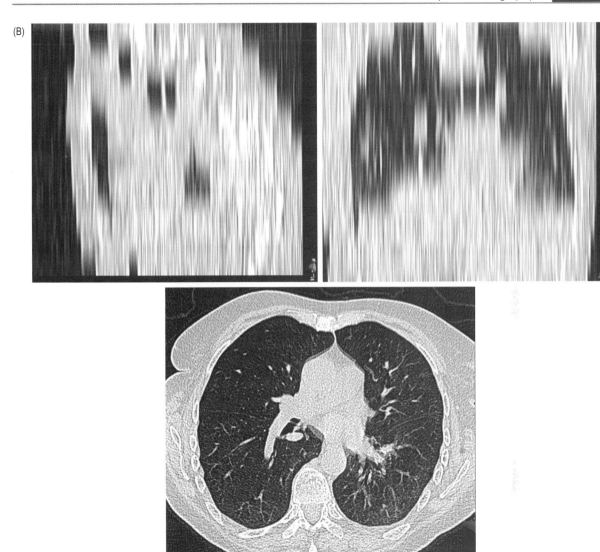

Fig. 4.14 (B) Anisotropic voxel data set. Whilst the x-y dimensions are equal, hence the same transaxial plane resolution, the z-axis values are different.

individual pixel varies (see Fig. 4.15). The signal-to-noise ratio (SNR) is governed by $M/\sqrt{M}$. Noise is therefore determined by $\sqrt{M}$, and directly affected by the photon flux. M is influenced by several factors:
Scanner:

- mA/scan time — increasing either or both increases the mAs and the number of photons (at a rate of $\sqrt{mA}$)

- Slice width — trade-off with reduced spatial resolution and increased partial volume effect
- kV — increased-kV photons have greater penetration (more are detected), but there is a trade-off with a reduction in contrast
- Matrix size/field of view — The more detectors that contribute to each pixel, the better the SNR. There is a trade-off with spatial resolution.

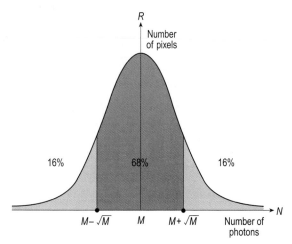

Fig. 4.15 The distribution of the number of X-ray photons absorbed in each pixel. R represents the number of pixels that absorb N photons. M is the average number of photons absorbed.

- Pitch — as pitch increases >1, noise increases.
Patient:
- Size — Larger patients require higher dose to achieve the same M as a smaller patient
- Amount of bones/metal in scan plane — can lead to photon starvation artefact (see below).
Electronic noise — This is inherent to the data acquisition system. Design and operation of the detector elements have bearings on the amount of intrinsic noise. Scatter also contributes to electronic noise

Structural noise — This relates to the processing of the collected data. Individual reconstruction algorithms have different effects on the underlying data and its representation in the final image. For instance, high-resolution kernels amplify noise as it is a high frequency.

Contrast

- mA
  - Lower mA, lower photon flux
- kV
  - Higher kV yields fewer low-energy photons which are important to detecting low-contrast objects
- Slice thickness
  - Partial volume effect
- Iterative reconstruction algorithms
  - Resolution is independent of dose and contrast

Artefacts

1. Motion
   Motion during scan acquisition adversely affects the reconstruction process. The moving structure occupies different voxels during the scan and causes artefacts. The main sources are:
   a. Cardiac motion in non-electrocardiography (ECG)-gated studies — addressed by ECG gating where necessary
   b. Breathing artefact — studies performed during breath-holding are optimal
   c. Patient movement — clear instructions to the patient reduces the chance of movement
2. High-attenuation objects
   a. Metal implants and dental amalgams give rise to streak artefacts that may obscure the area of interest. The streaks appear as dark and light lines emanating from the high-attenuation material. The effect is accentuated by motion. Small areas of bone or focal contrast medium can have a similar effect. Metal correction algorithms are standard and can be used to minimise the appearance of this artefact
   b. See Fig. 4.16
3. Photon starvation
   a. This is the result of insufficient photons reaching the detectors and can present as streaks or loss of contrast (see Fig. 4.17A). This is usually prevented with mA modulation, whereby the mA varies along the Z-axis according to the tolerances inferred by the patient's scout images.
   b. This can occur in patients who are very large in size and the mA required during modulation is beyond accepted tolerances (see Fig. 4.17B and C).
   c. Patients are not uniform in shape and the anteroposterior dimension is often less than width. mA modulation can be impaired if only one scout image is used to determine the required mA for a patient.
   d. The effects of photon starvation can be helped with the use of adaptive filtering, a technique that involves smoothing before reconstruction.
4. Beam hardening
   Lower-energy photons are absorbed more readily as the beam passes through the patient and are filtered out. The beam becomes harder (higher mean beam energy). This causes the attenuation coefficient and thus the CT number of a given tissue to decrease along the beam path. The reconstruction process assumes a homogeneous (i.e., monoenergetic) X-ray beam. The tissues towards the

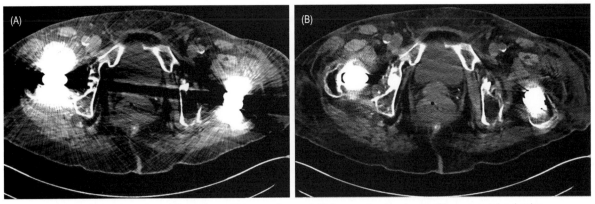

Fig. 4.16 Artefacts from bilateral metal hip prostheses. Initial reconstruction image (A); post-metal reduction algorithm (B).

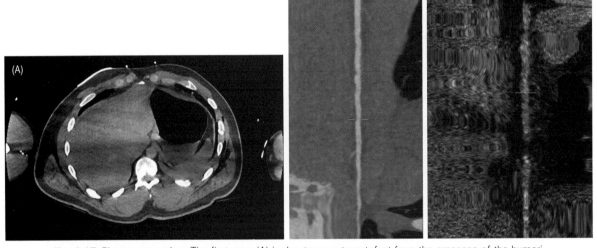

Fig. 4.17 Photon starvation. The first case (A) is due to an extra artefact from the presence of the humeri, leading to dark lines with limited contrast. The second case is due to a failure of mA modulation. (B) Reconstruction of a coronary artery in a normal study. (C) Reconstruction of a coronary artery for a study with significant photon starvation. There is significant noise with limited appreciation of anatomical detail.

centre of the patient are invariably crossed by hardened beams, whereas those nearer the surface are, for a significant part of the rotation time, crossed by photon beams that have not been filtered to the same extent. The result is that CT numbers are lower in the centre of the patient than they should be. This effect may be described as cupping. In some situations, it may also result in dark streaks in the image. It can be corrected to some extent by

a beam-hardening algorithm. The effect may also be reduced with the bow-tie filter that provides progressively increased filtration of the outer rays of the fan beam.

5. Ring

This is caused by a faulty detector in third-generation systems. The X-rays passing from the tube focus to a particular detector in the row of detectors trace out a circle as the gantry rotates about the patient (see Fig. 4.18). The

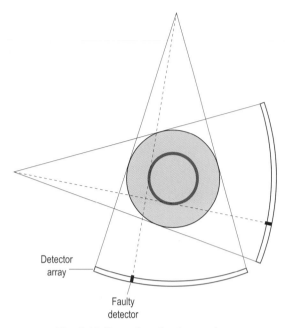

Fig. 4.18 Formation of a ring artefact.

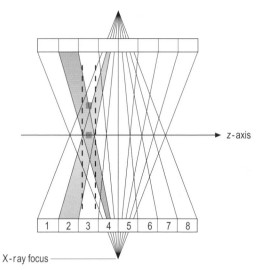

Fig. 4.19 Cone-beam effect. The effect of divergence in the reconstruction of out-of-plane slices for a multi-slice scanner; the dashed lines represent the plane reconstructed from detector 3.

CT numbers of the voxels that lie on that circle are calculated from the signal derived from that detector alone. Therefore, should that detector malfunction, the CT numbers in that ring will be incorrect and a light or dark ring will be seen in the image, depending on whether the detector is giving too low or too high a signal. It does not require a very big change in sensitivity of a single detector for a ring artefact to be visible. An operational feature of CT scanners is that, when they are switched on each day, automatic calibration programmes are run to check and adjust the calibration of the detectors to ensure that they provide a balanced response.
6. Partial volume effect

Each voxel represents the average attenuation coefficient of its components. A thin high-density structure that is only partially present in a voxel will increase the average value of that voxel and hence the thin structure appears larger. Low-contrast detail can also be lost as the difference is obscured during averaging. The partial volume effect is improved with decreased slice thickness.
7. Cone beam
   a. Multi-slice scanners — images are no longer in a single plane, but have a Z-axis component — partial volume effect. See Box 4.2.
   b. Compensated with reconstruction algorithms. If there is inadequate correction for this, an artefact is seen as a blurring at the boundaries between high-contrast details (e.g., at the boundary of bone and soft tissue).

BOX 4.2   Cone-Beam Effect

The object on the rotation axis (in Fig. 4.19) contributes to the ray sum of detector 2 and would be imaged on the slice plane defined by that detector, shown by the dashed line in the figure. However, the off-axis object that lies within the same slice plane contributes to the ray sums of detector 1 for the downward projection, and detectors 2 and 3 for the upward projection. In effect, the slice reconstructed from detector 2 relates to voxels within the shaded regions shown in the figure that would trace out a double cone in a full rotation.

The cone-beam effect becomes more significant with increased numbers of slices and with increasing total detector length. Cone-beam algorithms have had to be introduced to minimise the significance of this effect.

CT IMAGE PROCESSING

After the reconstruction process and CT image matrix generation, further processing can be performed.

Histogram processing is similar to the greyscale processing for X-rays. One technique is windowing (see Figs. 4.20–4.22) to make certain details more or less apparent. The 'windows' defined for lung, liver, soft

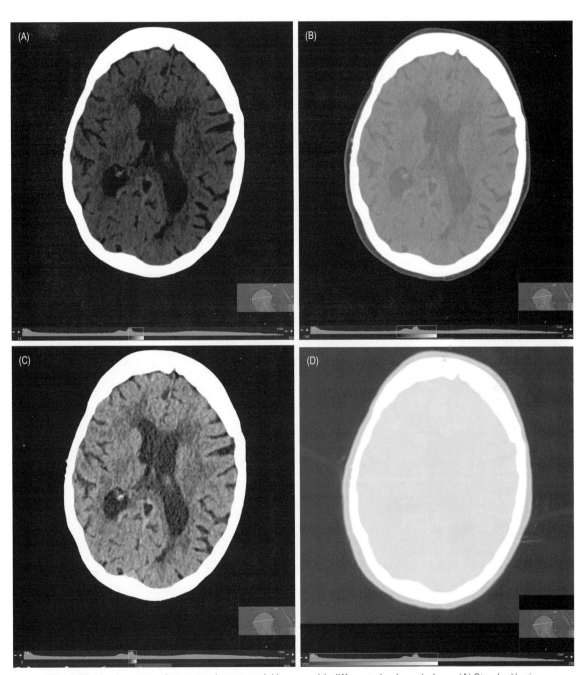

Fig. 4.20 Head computed tomography transaxial image, with different viewing windows. (A) Standard brain; (B) soft tissue; (C) stroke; (D) lung; (E) bone.

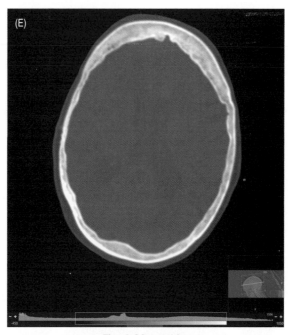

Fig. 4.20 cont'd.

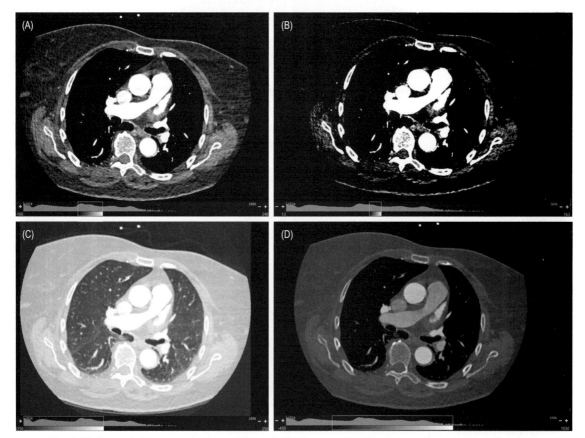

Fig. 4.21 Computed tomography images through the thorax, with different viewing windows. *A*, soft tissue; *B*, liver; *C*, lung; *D*, bone.

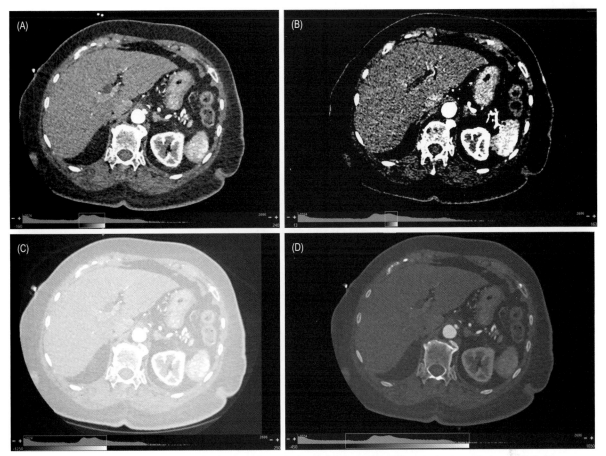

Fig. 4.22 Computed tomography images through the abdomen, with different viewing windows. (A) Soft tissue; (B) liver; (C) lung; (D) bone.

tissue, brain, and bone are often defined by pre-set look-up tables. These windows can have very different centres and widths as outlined in Table 4.2.

One of the major advantages of modern CT scanners is the multiplanar reformat (see Fig. 4.23). This enables any acquired dataset to be viewed in any plane. It is important to recognise that the dimensions of a rotating cube are not all the same (maximum difference of $\sqrt{3}:1$ in length). These discrepancies are accounted for by the imaging processing software allowing seamless multiplanar viewing for the isotropic dataset.

TABLE 4.2   CT Look-up Table

Name	Centre	Width
Soft Tissue	40	400
Lung	−500	1500
Liver	88	150
Bone	300	1500
CTPA	100	700
Blood	95	160
Stroke	65	20
Posterior Fossa	40	120
Supratentorial Brain	40	80

CTPA, Computed tomography pulmonary angiogram.

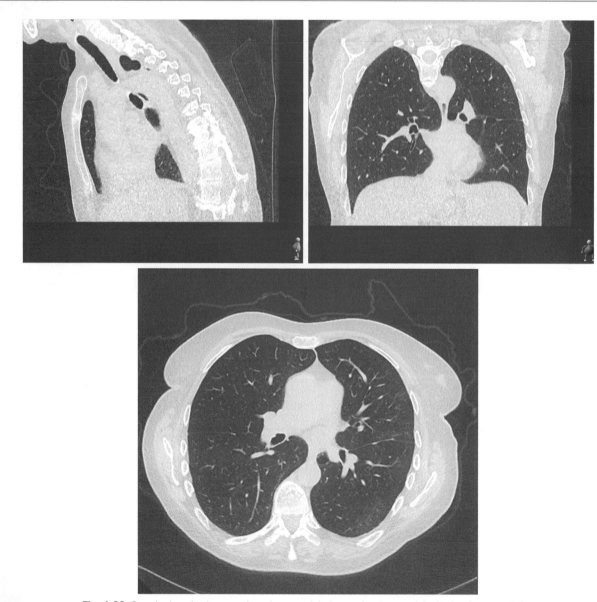

Fig. 4.23 Standard sagittal, coronal, and transaxial views of a dataset (clockwise from top left).

Another post-processing technique is that of the maximum intensity projection (MIP). Here the acquired dataset (at voxel sizes of 1 or 2 mm) can be processed and projected at any slice thickness above the minimum reconstructed thickness. The standard MIP is 10 mm but can be any value. This is used to make small structures more readily apparent (see Fig. 4.24).

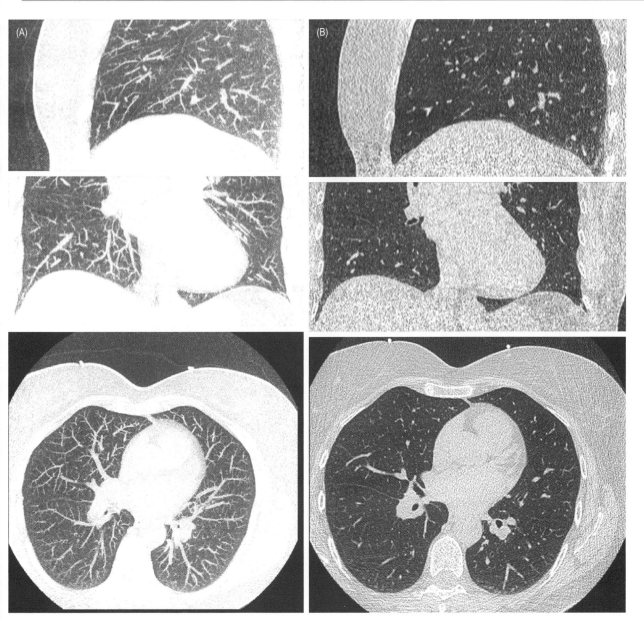

Fig. 4.24 (A) Maximum intensity projection (10 mm slice thickness) with the same centre voxel as (B) minimum intensity projection (1 mm reconstructed slice thickness).

A further common post-processing technique is that of volume renders. This enables certain voxel values in the image matrix to be hidden. This can make certain desired targets (e.g., blood vessels or bone) more readily apparent. This process uses alpha blending to make individual voxels more transparent relative to other voxels based on certain parameters (see Fig. 4.25). The parameters are becoming more complex, but two of the simpler ones are:

- Attenuation value threshold — All voxels with a certain value and above or below are displayed only
- Iso-surface — Only voxels of a certain value (or small range) are displayed

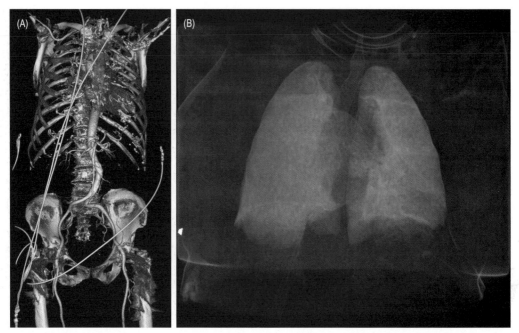

Fig. 4.25 (A) Volume render of a computed tomography angiogram using a simple threshold value for transparency (hence the bone, some muscles, and electrocardiography leads are displayed). (B) Volume render of the lungs using a threshold value designed to show inflation of both lungs.

ADDITIONAL CT CAPABILITIES

Cardiac CT/Gated imaging — The vastly improved temporal resolution (as a fast as 75 ms) and spatial resolution (<0.5 mm) of CT have allowed for the development of gated cardiac CT imaging (see Fig. 4.26). Previously, the motion of the heart during the cardiac cycle was too fast compared to the temporal resolution to allow for 'still' images to be acquired. The improved temporal resolution has allowed for imaging of the heart during fractions of the ECG cycle. The acquisition of images is coupled to the patient's ECG (see Figs. 4.27 and 4.28). Heart motion is minimal during diastole (often termed as 70% of the ECG cycle). There are different methods for acquisition:

Retrospective — The patient is irradiated throughout the cardiac cycle allowing for retrospective reconstruction at a desired point in the ECG cycle. This is a very high dose. The pitch is <1 so that there is overlap of the imaged heart during all phases of the ECG cycle.

Retrospective with dose modulation — In this variant of retrospective, the tube current is reduced when the ECG cycle is not in the acquisition window (usually reduced during systole, to facilitate diastole acquisition). The dose is less than full retrospective.

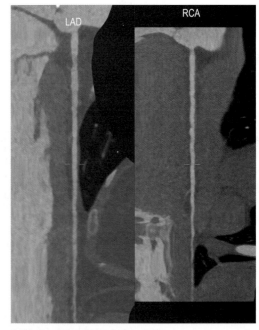

Fig. 4.26 Straightened reformat of two coronary arteries acquired from a dedicated CT coronary angiogram. *LAD*, Left anterior descending artery; *RCA*, right coronary artery.

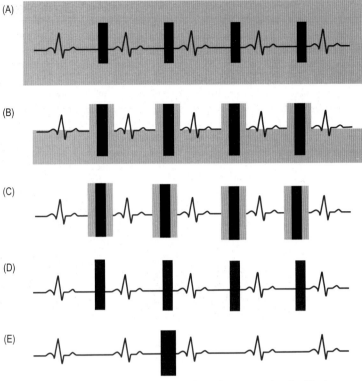

Fig. 4.27 Electrocardiogram gating. Lilac represents the tube current levels. Black represents the reconstructed acquisition window. (A) Retrospective, no modulation; (B) retrospective, tube modulation; (C) prospective, with padding; (D) prospective, no padding; (E) ultrahigh pitch.

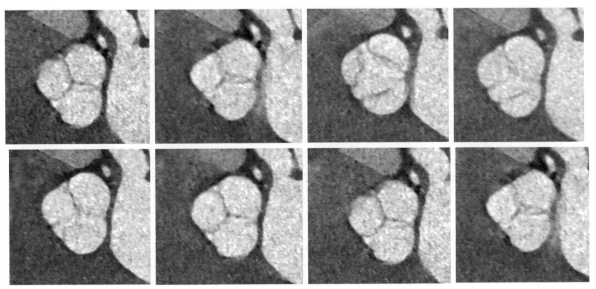

Fig. 4.28 Different phases of a cardiac cycle acquisition reconstructed showing the aortic valve open and closed.

Prospective — The patient's ECG is monitored with the timing of the cycle is anticipated and predicted. The scanner is triggered at a certain point in the cardiac cycle based on this prediction. For example, for diastolic acquisition, the timing is desired at 70% of the ECG cycle. Based on the ECG, the scanner is triggered at end systole (~45%) with the anticipation that diastole will occur as predicted. This is best achieved with steady heart rates, and can be prone to error (e.g., ectopic beats). The acquisition scan can be 'padded', whereby there is additional image acquisition before and after the desired point to help account for beat-beat variations.

In prospective imaging, a section of the heart (usually ~3 cm in the Z-axis) is imaged during one acquisition window. The patient table moves along the Z-axis in between each acquisition, similar to a 'step and shoot' acquisition. These 3-cm blocks are combined to form the final image (see Fig. 4.29).

Ultrahigh pitch — This utilises dual-source scanners and rapid table movement to cover the entire heart in 1 heartbeat. Each tube-detector array covers 90°. This technique needs low and steady heart beats (ideally <60 bpm).

Large detector width/cone-beam CT — The detector width in the Z-axis allows for full coverage of the heart in one acquisition (16 cm detector width). No table movement is necessary. One drawback is that increased image reconstruction is needed due to the increased cone-beam artefact compared to standard CT.

Angiography — Helical/spiral acquisition allows for the possibility of 3D imaging of vascular structures. These can be assessed during arterial or venous phases depending on contrast timings. The timing of contrast can obtained through either:

Bolus tracking — multiple single-slice images of the same region of interest are obtained during the administration of intravenous iodinated contrast. This region is often the aorta (ascending, descending, or abdominal depending on the study). After a certain HU threshold is exceeded in the region of interest by contrast-mixed blood (e.g., 160 HU), the complete scan begins with assumed good overall mixing of iodinated contrast.

Test bolus — a small volume of intravenous iodinated contrast is introduced. The HU profile of a region of interest (usually the aorta) is plotted using repeated single-slice acquisitions. The peak of the profile is used as the timing for the complete angiogram.

Isotropic voxels allow for true 3D imaging that can be viewed in multiple planes. The information available from CT is not limited to intraluminal information as in conventional fluoroscopic angiography.

Fluoroscopy — Real-time scanning for some interventional procedures. This is often a single-slice acquisition repeated multiple times. It is considered to be a high dose.

Ultrahigh pitch — Combination of dual X-ray sources to acquire two half datasets which are then combined to a single set.

Dual-energy CT — Utilising different kVp energies during the acquisition of a scan can yield further contrast. It harnesses the variant responses of the differing atomic numbers in the constituent atoms of a material to yield further contrast between these in a given voxel. This process provides conventional CT images (low kV, high kV, and mixed kV). It can generate material-specific images and varying colour maps. There are different approaches to the acquisition depending on scanner hardware specifications:

Single-source scanners — One mode is that of the fast kVp switch, whereby the X-ray tube source alternates rapidly during acquisition. Another involves consecutive repeat acquisitions of the same volume at different kVp.

Dual source — Each of the two separate X-ray tubes operates at different kVp, with matched detector arrays.

Detector-based spectral CT — This uses a double-layered detector array. The higher layer absorbs low-energy photons, whilst the deeper layer absorbs high-energy photons.

Applications:

Chest — Perfusion blood volume maps to indicate pulmonary emboli
See Fig. 4.30

Solid abdominal organs — Material-specific iodine images and virtual non-contrast datasets
Help distinguish high-density renal cysts vs renal malignancy
Distinguish thrombus vs tumour
Improved identification of lesion margins within liver/kidney
Renal calculus composition

Bone — Virtual subtraction of calcium to demonstrate marrow oedema

Artefact reduction — Can reduce beam-hardening artefacts from metal implants

CT perfusion — This is a technique to enable characterisation of blood delivery in tissue. It is most often used in stroke imaging (see Fig. 4.31). There are a few steps in the process:

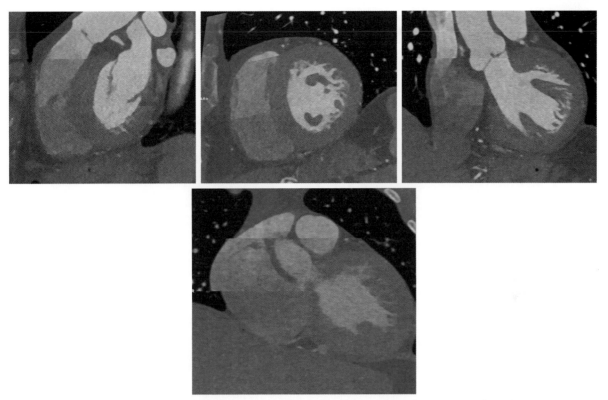

Fig. 4.29 Reconstructed heart images from 4 'stitched together' datasets. The top row is from the same acquisition with good alignment. The bottom image show how beat-beat variation can distort the data volume.

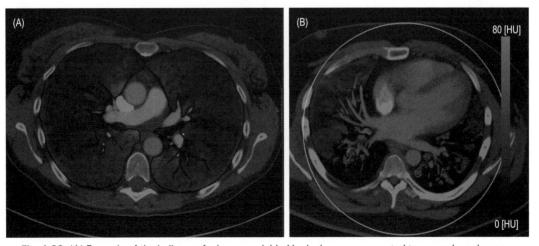

Fig. 4.30 (A) Example of the iodine perfusion map yielded in dual-energy computed tomography pulmonary angiogram *(CTPA)*, viewed with a colour map. (B) Example of perfusion defects in a CTPA (black areas).

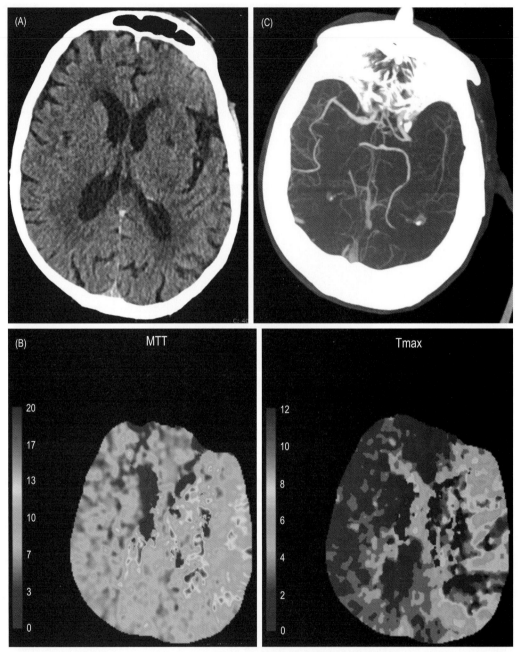

Fig. 4.31 (A) Unenhanced image of the brain with defects on the left (including, but not limited to the insular cortex, frontal cortex, and lentiform nucleus). (B) Colour maps of the mean transit time (*MTT*) and time to peak *(Tmax)* showing increases in the left. (C) Maximum intensity projection of a computed tomography angiogram showing occlusion of the left middle cerebral artery.

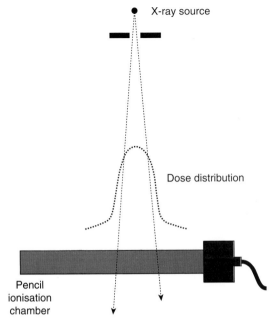

Fig. 4.32 An ionisation chamber. The charge emitted from the chamber is proportional to the area under the dose-distribution curve.

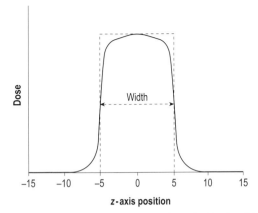

Fig. 4.33 Dose profile of X-ray beam along the Z-axis with an ideal square beam profile (dashed line).

1. Unenhanced scan of the organ of interest
2. Contrast administration — Iodine disperses to extracellular space as well as intravascular compartment
3. Dynamic image acquisition — Multiple repeated acquisitions of the volume of interest
4. Model the variation in attenuation of each individual voxel over time — Identify regions of delayed contrast enhancement indicating ischaemia

CT photon counting — This is a newly emerging technology at the time of writing. The detectors in these scanners can quantify the individual photon kV at each detection. This information can then be used to yield multiple datasets similar to dual-energy CT, but without the additional dose.

DOSE

CT is overall a high-dose technique. Whilst the dose for some techniques has reduced over the years (e.g., low-dose thorax CT used in lung cancer screening), the dose for other examinations remains high (e.g., trauma scans, multiphase cardiac CT).

The dose for a given CT scan is usually quantified in terms of dose length product (DLP). There are a few processes before such a value is obtained.

The first aspect in the process is the dosimeter, which enables dose measurement. This is usually a pencil ionisation chamber (see Fig. 4.32). The pencil ionisation chamber is a small air-filled container (8 mm wide, 100 mm long). It measures electric charge caused by the passage of X-rays through the chamber. This charge is proportional to the amount of incident radiation.

The CT dose index (CTDI) represents the measured dose (in mGy) from a single gantry rotation. International standards for CTDI are used to compare the dose exposure for different scanners. Fig. 4.33 shows the typical dose profile along the Z-axis, for a beam collimated to a width of 10 mm. There are comparable areas between the ideal square beam profile and the true dose profile. The peak value is the maximum absorbed dose in the scan plane, and is dependent on kV, mAs, and filtration rather than slice width.

$$CTDI = \int D(z).dz/T$$

where $D(z)$ = dose, T = slice width (along the Z-axis)

- Equivalent to the area under the dose profile

CTDI$_w$ represents the weighted CTDI. This is derived to account for variation in dose across the cross-section of a patient. The dose at the periphery is higher than at the centre. This value is determined by use of phantoms (see Fig. 4.34):
- Head — 16 cm diameter
- Body — 32 cm diameter

Ionisation chambers are placed at central and peripheral locations to determine relative CTDI values.

$$CTDI_w = {}^1\!/_3 CTDI_{centre} + {}^2\!/_3 CTDI_{periphery}$$

$$CTDI_{vol} = CTDI_w/pitch$$

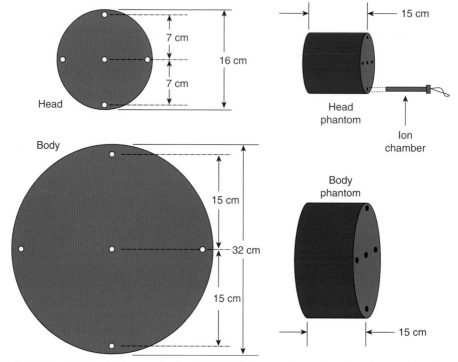

Fig. 4.34 A view of a 'head' phantom (top) and a 'body' phantom (bottom). Dimensions and location of the ionisation chamber holes are shown. Diameters of the holes are typically 1 cm and should be drilled to match the outer diameter of the ionisation chamber.

where $CTDI_{vol}$ represents the average absorbed dose within the scanned volume.

CTDI is useful for describing the dose efficiency of a scan protocol and for comparisons between scan models. However, it is less useful for a comparison of doses to individual patients, because attention also has to be given to the length of scan and to the number of times a particular region might be scanned (e.g., pre- and post-intravenous contrast administration). The DLP, measured in mGy.cm, is defined as:

$$DLP = CTDI_{vol} . L$$

where L is the total scan length. The length may be estimated from the number of rotations multiplied by collimated length and pitch.

Effective dose (E) can be derived from DLP, based upon conversion coefficients. The unit is the millisievert (mSv) and is equivalent to J/kg. The conversion factor is based on body location, with radiosensitive organs such as the gonads having a high conversion factor.

$$E = \sum \omega_T . H_T$$

- ω_T = tissue weighting
- H_T = Equivalent dose to tissue
  Factors affecting dose:
- mAs:
  - Milliamperage and time combined, determines the quantity of incident photons during the scan
  - Dose is directly proportional to mAs (doubling mAs doubles dose)
- kVp:
  - Peak kilovoltage
  - Dose is proportional to $(kVp)^2$
- Pitch
  - Dose is inversely proportional to pitch (doubling pitch, halves dose)
- Collimation
  - Controls the slice width of the X-ray beam
  - The penumbra of the beam should not fall on the detectors
- Patient centring
  - Patient must be positioned in isocentre of gantry, otherwise dose and noise are increased.
  - If the patient is placed closer to the tube than the isocentre, a larger scout radiograph is produced.

The automated tube current modulation is increased incorrectly assuming a larger patient.

Dose Optimisation

- Tube current modulation
  - Based on the scout image/topogram
  - Varies tube current used based on the attenuation values only on the Z-axis
  - Areas of high attenuation (e.g., across shoulders) require and receive more mA than lower attenuation areas (e.g., mid-thorax)
- Optimal tube voltage
  - Vary voltage based on patient body mass index
  - Smaller patients can be imaged at 80 or 100 kV compared with 120 kV for large patients
  - Screening studies (CT colonography, lung cancer screening) can tolerate lower kV and noisier images as they are looking for discrete incidental nodules or polyps
  - CT examinations of kidney, ureter, or bladder can have lower kV as these studies look for high-contrast calculi
- Patient centring and positioning
  - Centre patient appropriately to maximise the accuracy of the scout image
  - Where possible, remove arms from the exposure
- Noise-reducing image reconstruction algorithms
  - Hybrid iterative reconstruction and FBP algorithms allow noise and dose reduction without significant increase in computational power

- Limited to new scanners
- Scan range/mode
  - Limit a scan to region of interest only
  - Judicious use of multiphase scanning (pre-contrast, arterial, venous phase scans)
  - Use of prospective or ultrahigh-pitch dual-source acquisition modes in cardiac CT rather than retrospective

FURTHER READING

Hansen M, others. Computed tomography (CT) perfusion in abdominal cancer: technical aspects. *Diagnostics*. 2013;3: 261–270.

Konstas AA, others. Theoretic basis and technical implementations of CT perfusion in acute ischemic stroke, part 1: theoretic basis. *AJNR Am J Neuroradiol*. 2009;30:662–668.

Mayo-Smith WW, others. How I do it: managing radiation dose in CT. *Radiology*. 2014;273:657–672.

Patino M, others. Material separation using dual-energy CT: current and emerging applications. *Radiographics*. 2016;36:1087–1105.

Schardt P, others. New x-ray tube performance in computed tomography by introducing the rotating envelope tube technology. *Med Phys*. 2004;31:2699–2706.

Seeram E. *Computed Tomography: Physical Principles, Clinical Applications, and Quality Control*. 4th ed. St. Louis: Elsevier Health Sciences; 2015.

5

Nuclear Imaging

CHAPTER CONTENTS

THE GAMMA CAMERA

The goal of radionuclide imaging, or nuclear medicine, is to image the distribution of the radiopharmaceutical within the patient using the gamma radiation that it emits. The imaging device used to achieve this is known as a gamma camera.

The main components of a gamma camera are:

- A collimator
- A large-area radiation detector
- Electronics for radiation detection
- Electronics for signal processing
- A computer for image display and data storage

The first four components are generally grouped in the detector head, as shown in Fig. 5.1. The original basic design for the gamma camera detector head was formulated in the mid-1950s and has undergone little change since then, although there have considerable improvements in individual components. The early gamma cameras were analogue devices, but modern cameras are digital devices, and there will be a further generational step forward in this respect in the next few years.

Collimator

After a patient has been injected with the radiopharmaceutical, they are emitting gamma rays in all directions. To obtain an interpretable image, some correlation must be achieved between the origin of the emission within the patient and its position within the image. The collimator establishes a linear relationship between the origin and the point of contact on the surface of the radiation detector (i.e., only photons travelling directly perpendicular to the surface are allowed through the collimator).

The most common type is the parallel-hole collimator, in which hole shapes may be round, square, triangular, or more typically, hexagonal. Collimators are generally made of lead because of its high linear attenuation coefficient; the lead between two adjacent holes is called the septum. A collimator for imaging technetium-99m ($^{99}Tc^m$) will have tens of thousands of holes each of about 1–2 mm in diameter. The thickness of the septa is determined by the energy of the gamma photons emitted by the radiopharmaceutical. The septa must be thick enough to absorb most of the photons incident upon them. Thus, collimators designed for ^{131}I (364 keV) have thicker septa than those designed for $^{99}Tc^m$ (140 keV).

Parallel-hole collimators are usually classified as low, medium, or high energy according to the maximum photon energy with which they can be used satisfactorily. Most cameras will have a range of collimator pairs (i.e., low-energy general purpose [LEGP] and low-energy high resolution [LEHR]) which are optimised for use with gamma emissions from $^{99}Tc^m$. Most departments will also have at least one of medium-energy general purpose (MEGP) which are optimised for emissions around 250 keV and high-energy general purpose (HEGP) which are for emissions over 350 keV. If the septa are too thin, there is an increased probability of penetration by gamma photons that are not travelling parallel to the axes of the holes, a phenomenon known as septal penetration. These

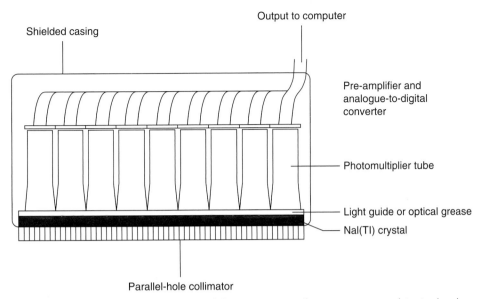

Fig. 5.1 Simplified schematic diagram of the components of a gamma camera detector head.

result in degradation of image quality due to reduced contrast and spatial resolution.

Parallel-hole collimators are made using a few different methods:

- Crimped lead foil sheets
- Drilled lead block
- Casting from molten lead

Drilled or cast collimators are the optimal methods of construction because no gaps are left in the septa, thus giving better image contrast and spatial resolution. Foil collimators are less expensive but have gaps where the sheets are glued together, leading to an increased probability of septal penetration. Failure of the glue lines can also lead to sagging of the foils as the camera head rotates.

Modern collimators are heavy and generally require mechanical assistance for fitting to the gamma camera. MEGP and HEGP collimators can be 80–115 kg each. Different manufacturers have a variety of devices for storing and fitting the collimators. These include carts and automatic trays built in to the camera bed. The removal and installation of the collimators may be done automatically or semi-automatically, where some operator intervention is required. This is particularly important for multihead cameras where any physical intervention required must be repeated multiple times depending on the number of detector heads.

Fig. 5.2 shows the range of collimator designs which are typically available. In general, other types of collimators

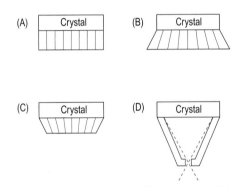

Fig. 5.2 A selection of typical collimator types: (A) parallel hole, (B) diverging hole, (C) converging hole, (D) pinhole.

are much less frequently used than parallel-hole collimators. Only pinhole and converging collimators have any practical utility in modern systems.

The pinhole is a single-hole collimator that is used to produce magnified views of small objects (e.g., thyroid). It consists of a small (3–5 mm) hole at the apex of a leaded cone. Like a pinhole camera, magnification is achieved if the pinhole-object distance is less than the detector-pinhole distance. The use of a pinhole means that photons interact with a much larger area of the detector than would be the case with a parallel-hole collimator. The downside is that the resultant image is inverted and flipped, which may cause complications with anatomical labelling if the image is incorrectly labelled.

Converging collimators give a magnified image, and this may be useful when the object is much smaller than the field of view. The image size depends on the distance between the object and the collimator. The disadvantage of these is that the extremities of the patient, such as the arms, may not be included in the image and this can lead to the creation of truncation artefacts in tomographic images. Some manufacturers are now producing 'variable focus' collimators which are converging in the centre to focus on target organs, often the heart, but alter as you move away from the centre to become parallel-hole at the edges. This magnifies the target organ but avoids creating truncation artefacts. However, proprietary image reconstruction software is required to deal with the specific geometry of the collimators.

Radiation Detector

The collimator is fitted to the front of the detector head which contains the radiation detector and associated equipment. Typically, the detector is a large-area NaI(Tl) scintillation crystal — a single crystal of sodium iodide doped with around 10% thallium. NaI is a fluorescent material which converts the energy absorbed into visible light. The crystals are typically 6—13 mm thick with most systems now using a crystal of around 9 mm. This provides the optimal combination of stopping power for the incident gamma rays whilst minimising self-absorption of the generated light and the probability of scatter of the incident radiation.

The original detector crystals were circular with a diameter of just over 30 cm. However, the ability to grow large, single crystals for NaI has been developed, and crystals are now rectangular and around 60 × 50 cm. This is large enough to cover the entire width of the patient so imaging of the entire patient can be achieved quickly in a minimum number of images. Sodium iodide is hygroscopic, so the crystal is hermetically sealed in aluminium with a transparent window adjacent to one face so that the light can escape. The inner faces of the aluminium containment are coated in a reflective compound to ensure maximum light output.

Photons that reach the crystal may interact or pass through without interaction. At 140 keV, most photons that interact do so through the photoelectric effect with the remainder undergoing Compton scattering. Gamma photon energy is absorbed through photoelectrons and Compton recoil electrons to create a scintillation. Each scintillation contains around 5000 light photons and has a very short decay time of around 600 ns.

Photomultiplier Tubes

Behind the crystal is an array of 30—100 photomultiplier tubes (PMTs) that detect the visible light. An optical glass light guide or layer of silicone grease is used to maintain good optical contact between the exit window of the detector and the entrance window of the PMTs.

The PMT is a vacuum tube that detects a very small amount of light, such as that produced in a scintillation, and converts and amplifies it into a measurable electrical signal. The incident light energy releases electrons from a **photocathode.** For optimal performance, the peak light response of the photocathode should be matched to the wavelength of the light produced by the crystal. As shown in Fig. 5.3, inside the tube are a series of **dynodes** that are held at increasing positive potential to each other by a high-voltage supply. The electrons are accelerated by the potential differences and gain kinetic energy. They also generate new electrons which allow the PMT to act as an electron amplifier and a relatively large amount of negative charge, around a billion times larger than the original signal, is collected at the **anode**. This generates a current pulse which forms the output signal.

The amplification (gain) of a PMT, and hence the amount of charge produced at the anode, is strongly influenced by the high voltage. The gain of each PMT must be matched to that of the other tubes in the array and this requires constant fine adjustment of the high voltage applied to each. One method of gain stabilisation is to periodically feed a fixed amount of light into each PMT, monitor the amount of charge produced at the anode, and adjust the high voltage as necessary. LEDs act as a stable source of light and this is conducted to the PMTs by fibre-optic cables.

Pulse Arithmetic

The amount of light received by a particular PMT depends on the inverse square of the distance from the scintillation in the crystal to that PMT. This helps in the calculation of event position. Each PMT produces a pulse whose magnitude depends on the amount of light it receives. This helps in the calculation of event energy. The pulse heights

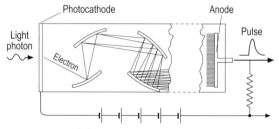

Fig. 5.3 Schematic of a photomultiplier tube.

from the PMTs carry information about the position and energy of the incident gamma photon. Thus, the pulse arithmetic to determine these is carried out on the digitised signals from the printed circuit board on the output of each PMT. This contains a pre-amplifier and the analogue-to-digital converters.

Assume that there are n PMTs of designation i. The X and Y coordinates of the scintillation are given by:

$$X = \frac{\sum_{i=0}^{n} v_i x_i}{\sum_{i=0}^{n} v_i} \quad Y = \frac{\sum_{i=0}^{n} v_i y_i}{\sum_{i=0}^{n} v_i}$$

where v_i is the height of the voltage pulse from the ith PMT (in volts). X and Y have the same distance units as the individual x_i and y_i.

The absorbed energy is proportional to:

$$Z = \sum_{i=0}^{n} v_i$$

The X and Y coordinates calculated are those of the centroid of the signals from the PMTs. X and Y position calculations are independent of the gamma energy. Thus, a 140-keV photon and a 364-keV photon that are completely absorbed at the same position in the crystal generate different values of v_i and hence Z, but identical values of X and Y.

Pulse Height Analysis

This is the process by which unwanted, scattered radiation is excluded from the final image. As shown in Fig. 5.4, a

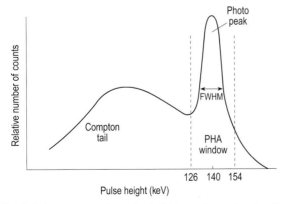

Fig. 5.4 A representative pulse height spectrum showing the relative frequency of pulses of differing heights. *FWHM*, full width at half maximum; *PHA*, pulse height analyser.

fixed-width energy window is used centred on the photopeak within which the events will be accepted to create the image. Because of the finite energy resolution of the detector, there is some overlap between the photopeak and the Compton band. This means that some unscattered photons will be rejected and some scattered photons accepted. The use of a 20% acceptance window (i.e., photopeak energy ± 10%), also rejects the occasional high Z value due to high-energy background radiation or the random coincident detection of more than one gamma photon in the crystal. Narrower photopeak windows will exclude more scatter but will reduce sensitivity as less photopeak events are accepted.

Multiple windows can be defined for radioisotopes with multiple gamma emissions. However, there will be down scatter from the Compton band of the highest-energy emissions into the photopeak windows of the lower energy windows. This must be considered when deciding which windows to use, and corrections may be required to account for this.

Computer Processing

The position and energy of accepted events after pulse height analysis are passed to the acquisition computer to facilitate creation of the final image. These are provided by the manufacturer as part of the gamma camera package and provide software to control the acquisition, display, and processing of the images. These are often linked to further computers which allow more complex post-processing and analysis of the images to improve the information available to the person reporting the images. These systems may be provided by the gamma camera manufacturer or by specialist third-party providers.

The acquisition camera will also contain a large-capacity hard disc to store the acquired data for. The capacity of these will normally allow for the storage of a few weeks or months of patient data. However, these will generally also be sent to a digital picture archiving and communication systems (PACS) or other storage systems to allow permanent archiving of the data.

Solid-State Detectors

In recent years, a small number of 'direct digital detection' systems have become available commercially. These replace the scintillation crystal and PMTs with a solid-state detector, generally of cadmium-zinc-telluride (CZT). This can improve the energy resolution by a factor of around 2 in comparison to the traditional design. This improves the exclusion of scattered radiation and hence leads to improved image contrast.

There are technical difficulties in producing large-area detectors with CZT, so their greatest foothold in the marketplace has so far come in dedicated cardiac systems. These use small field-of-view L-shaped detectors to get close to the chest and can acquire adequate data faster than conventional camera systems. Dedicated tomographic systems are also now available using multiple, rotating CZT detectors, but these are still rare due to their lack of flexibility, as they can only be used for tomographic imaging.

Other Components of the Gamma Camera

Many modern gamma camera systems have dual detector heads as this increases the flexibility of the system and allows the faster acquisition of the required amount of data. There are also single-headed systems available which can be useful where space is restricted as these tend to have a smaller physical footprint. Triple-headed, dedicated neuroimaging systems are also available, although these are less common due to their very specific purpose and lack of flexibility.

Gantry

The detector heads are mounted on a gantry which supports the heads and allows a full range of movement around the patient. Many systems now use a circular gantry arrangement as this allows for maximum flexibility in positioning and is highly suited to tomographic imaging, as will be described later. Most circular gantries also use slip-ring technologies where signals and power are passed from the static section of the gantry to the rotating section using brushes and contact bars. These allow the gantry to rotate up to 540° before the system must be reset to the origin position.

The detector heads will generally also rotate on their individual mounting points to allow the acquisition of oblique views and can also move radially to increase or reduce the distance between the detector head and the patient. Most systems will also allow a small amount of lateral motion of the heads.

Patient Table

Usually, the patient table comprises a base unit securely mounted to the floor with a long, thin but very strong pallet on the top for the patient to lie upon. The table will have hydraulic functions to allow the height to be changed, dropping low to the floor to allow safe patient access, and driving up to the required height for optimal imaging.

Key features of the pallet include:
- It should be manufactured from carbon fibre or similar material which has low attenuation characteristics (<10% at 140 keV).
- It should support a 200-kg patient without significant sagging.
- It should be of narrow width ($\sim$35 cm) to allow the detector heads as close to the patient as possible.
- It should have restraint straps to keep the patient stable and safe.
- Ideally it should also have a narrower head restraint for brain imaging.

In practice, although the bed may have a weight limit suitable for very large patients, the narrowness of the pallet means that it may be very difficult to get the patient in a stable, safe position for imaging. In cases where this is suspected, the patient should be tested on the table prior to injection so that they are not exposed to a radiation dose when no useable images may be obtained.

Some manufacturers also now incorporate other functions into the structure of the patient table. These include collimator storage trays to allow the use of automated collimator exchange systems. Automated quality-control systems are also available where sealed sources of specific radionuclides are stored in shielded compartments within the table and can be exposed for the acquisition of routine quality-control checks. Appropriate radiation protection safeguards must be in place if these are used.

Control Systems

Most systems will have control panels mounted on the gantry which allow control of the movement of the detector heads and patient table and the starting and stopping of image acquisition. These are generally on both sides of the gantry and may also be on the front and back to allow the maximum flexibility for staff in their control of the system. Some systems also have flat-panel, touchscreen control panels mounted on a long arm which can be moved around the system and allow control of functions such as the automated collimator changers. These may also double as DVD players and are very useful for keeping children entertained during scans.

Fig. 5.5 shows an image of a typical modern dual-detector gamma camera system displaying many of the features just mentioned.

REAL-TIME SIGNAL CORRECTIONS

Corrections to the calculated position and energy signals for spatial linearity and energy are applied in real time. These address fundamental variations in the calculated

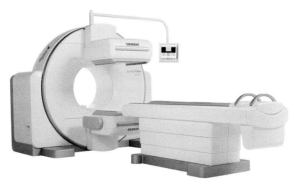

Fig. 5.5 Image of a typical modern dual-head gamma camera system. (Credit Siemens Healthcare Ltd.)

signals due to the camera design and construction. These must be corrected prior to displaying the image or incorrectly positioned events will be viewed. Fig. 5.6 shows a schematic of the processing carried out on the signals from the PMTs prior to their transfer to the display system.

Spatial non-linearity is caused by systematic mis-positioning of events which tend to be shifted towards the centre of the nearest PMT. This is due to the circular shape of the PMTs which leaves gaps between them no matter how tightly packed. Events which occur in the gaps will tend to be shifted toward the nearest PMT. This leads to a distortion where the image of a straight line appears 'wavy' as events are pulled into incorrect positions.

Energy varies with position due to factors such as variation in light production within the crystal, light transmission to the photocathode, light detection, and residual PMT gain. This leads to a distortion where an image of a uniform distribution of activity appears to have 'hot spots' within it corresponding to the positions of the PMTs.

As both these distortions are a result of the physical construction of the camera detector, they do not vary in time and can be measured in the factory prior to final construction. Look-up tables can be created which store the required corrections to the positional and energy signals for events occurring at any point in the crystal. These corrections can then be applied to the signals in real time.

GAMMA CAMERA PERFORMANCE PARAMETERS AND QUALITY CONTROL

Spatial Resolution

Spatial resolution is a measure of the camera's ability to distinguish between small radioactive sources that are close to each other. It is not a measure of the smallest thing visible in the image; it is the distance necessary between two objects for them to be resolved as separate.

It is defined as the full width at half maximum (FWHM) of the count profile when a line or point source of radioactivity is imaged as shown in Fig. 5.7. In the first case, the curve is the line spread function (LSF), while in the second case it is the point spread function (PSF). The units of

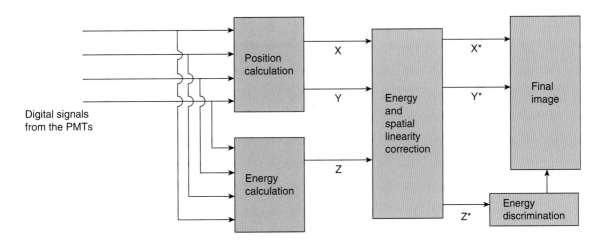

X*, Y* and Z* are the corrected positional and energy signals

Fig. 5.6 Schematic of the processing circuitry through which the signals from the photomultiplier tubes (PMTs) are passed prior to display of the image.

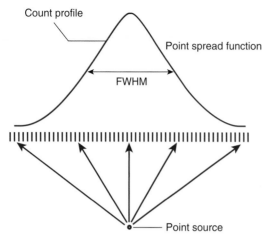

Fig. 5.7 Diagram of the formation of a point spread function for a parallel-hole collimator.

FWHM are those of distance (mm or cm); the smaller the FWHM, the better the resolution.

The overall spatial resolution of a gamma camera (the system spatial resolution) depends on the following factors:

- Intrinsic spatial resolution of the gamma camera
- Spatial resolution of the collimator
- Patient motion
- Pixelation effects

Intrinsic Resolution

The intrinsic spatial resolution R_I is the limiting value achievable by the detector and the electronics. It depends on many inter-related factors including:

Energy and Linearity Correction of the X, Y and Z Values Produced by Each Scintillation. This improves both spatial and energy resolution.

Photoelectron Range in the Sodium Iodide Crystal. This defines the dimensions of the volume of crystal from which light is emitted in a given scintillation. However, it is generally less than 1 mm and therefore negligible compared with other effects.

Gamma Photon Energy. The greater the gamma energy, the greater the number of scintillation photons reaching a particular PMT and so the smaller their relative statistical variation.

Collection of Scintillation Light. Optimising light collection gives better spatial resolution. Collection is improved by good optical coupling and PMT shape — square or hexagonal PMTs cover a greater area of crystal than circular ones.

Detection of Scintillation Light. More efficient PMT photocathodes improve spatial resolution by increasing the number of electrons released thus reducing relative statistical variation.

Number and Size of PMTs. A larger number of PMTs improves spatial resolution due to better sampling of the light, provided that the number of scintillation photons per PMT is acceptable.

Thresholding the PMT Voltage Signal. Only PMT signals above a minimum voltage are used for the calculation of position values. This eliminates very noisy signals.

Thickness of the NaI(Tl) Detector Crystal. The thicker the crystal, the worse the spatial resolution for two reasons:

- Greater variation in depth at which scintillations occur — leads to variations in light distribution among the PMTs
- Greater probability of multiple Compton scatter

The intrinsic resolution of a typical modern system at 140 keV is typically 2.5—4 mm FWHM.

There is a fundamental trade-off in the design of the conventional gamma camera detector head which must be considered at this stage. To maximise the intrinsic resolution, you wish to maximise the light detected by the nearest PMT, and so a thin light guide is optimal. However, to optimise the spatial linearity, you want to spread the light signal between the maximum number of PMTs, and hence a thicker light guide is best.

As was shown above, linearity is a fixed phenomenon and can be measured and corrected for, but resolution cannot be recovered once it is lost. Therefore, in practical systems, the light guide is minimised to maximise the intrinsic resolution achievable, and linearity is corrected using the real-time circuitry. This is why many systems now no longer include a light guide and the PMTs are coupled directly to the back of the crystal using an optical grease.

Collimator Resolution

For a parallel-hole collimator, spatial resolution R_C is given by:

$$R_C = d\left(1 + \left(b/h\right)\right)$$

where d is the hole diameter, h is the hole length, and b is the source distance. The collimator resolution is thus improved by using a collimator with long holes as this minimises the second term in the equation.

For many manufacturers, their LEGP and LEHR collimators will have identical hole sizes and septal thickness. The only difference will be in the thickness of the collimator, which determines the hole length. This simplifies the production process as the same mould can be used for both collimators with only the quantity of lead used determining the type of collimator produced.

System Resolution

The system resolution R_S is given by the sum of squares of the components which contribute to it. R_I and R_C are the most significant and the others contribute only minimally. Therefore:

$$R_S^2 = R_I^2 + R_C^2$$

Thus, the system spatial resolution is worse than that of any single component and the collimator is the dominant factor. The system resolution of a typical modern gamma camera measured in air on the collimator face will be around 5–7 mm. This will degrade with distance from the camera face and depth of tissue.

Modulation Transfer Function

The Fourier transform of the LSF or PSF is the modulation transfer function (MTF). The MTF is a complete mathematical description of the resolution properties of an imaging system. It gives the fraction of an object's contrast that is recorded by the imaging system as a function of the spatial frequency of the object.

The ideal MTF would have a response of 1 at all spatial frequencies (i.e., all frequencies are perfectly handled by the system). However, this is virtually impossible as even the human visual system cannot approach that goal.

The poorer the resolution of a system, the closer the curve will be to the origin, whereas systems with better resolution will produce MTF curves which are closer to the top right corner of the plot, nearer to the idealised perfect response. This can be seen in Fig. 5.8.

Sensitivity

The sensitivity of a gamma camera is a measure of the number of counts recorded, per unit time, when a fixed source of activity is placed in front of the detector. This is generally measured in units of counts per second per megabecquerel (cps/MBq). This will generally be measured for each collimator pair.

Uniformity

The uniformity of a gamma camera is described by analysing how uniform an image of a uniform distribution of radioactivity is. This is affected by the variations in both linearity and energy which results in it being the

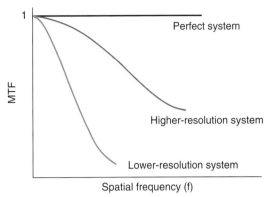

Fig. 5.8 Diagram of the modulation transfer functions (MTFs) obtained from a perfect imaging system and higher- and lower-resolution imaging systems.

fundamental performance parameter of the system. The uniformity of the system must be within the allowed limits before any patient imaging is carried out and therefore must be checked on at least a daily basis.

Energy Resolution

The calculated absorbed energy Z of an event depends on the energy of the gamma photon emitted from the patient and the fraction that is absorbed in the crystal:
- If the photon interacts with the crystal via the photoelectric effect, all its energy is absorbed (through the photoelectron)
- If the photon suffers one or more Compton interactions in the crystal (with the singly or multiply scattered photon escaping from the crystal), only part of its energy will be absorbed (through one or more recoil electrons)
- If a photon undergoes one or more Compton interactions followed by a photoelectric interaction, its full energy is again absorbed (through one or more recoil electrons and a photoelectron)

Fig. 5.9 shows these plotted for $^{99}Tc^m$ in an ideal situation and what is seen in reality. In the ideal situation, the unscattered radiation appears as a *delta* function at the 140-keV energy of the incident gamma rays with a continuous discrete tail at lower energies where the gamma rays have undergone Compton interactions within the patient or crystal. In reality, due to the energy variations described above, the unscattered radiation spreads into a photopeak around the primary energy with a continuous tail known as the Compton band. The inflection point where the photopeak and Compton band meet is sometimes referred to as the Compton edge.

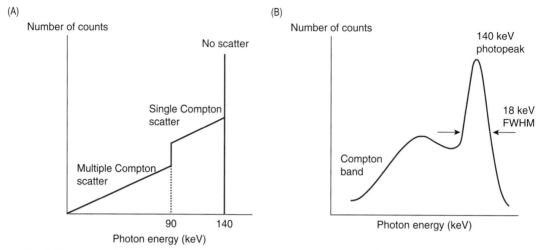

Fig. 5.9 Diagram of the energy spectrum obtained from technetium-99m in (A) an idealised situation and (B) a real situation.

Theoretically, the photopeak should be very narrow. However, it has a measurable width. This is usually expressed as the FWHM of the photopeak.

The energy resolution is given as a percentage by:

$$\frac{\text{FWHM (keV)}}{\text{Energy at peak (keV)}} \times 100$$

In the example in Fig. 5.9, the energy resolution is:

$$\frac{18 \text{ (keV)}}{140 \text{ (keV)}} \times 100 = 12.9\%$$

Most modern gamma camera systems produce an energy resolution of around 9%.

Count Rate Performance

Due to the finite processing time of each event within the system, gamma cameras do not produce a linear response between the recorded count rate and the activity being imaged. The response is linear up to a point but then, as the activity increases, events will be lost as their occurrence overlaps with the processing time of the previous event. However, although the event is lost from inclusion within the image, it extends the time during which events cannot be recorded, known as the 'dead time'. On modern systems, the point at which the relationship deviates from the linear lies at an activity of 70–90 MBq. Beyond this, as the activity increases, the count rate will drop away until it reaches a plateau value at the maximum achievable count rate. It will then drop away until the recorded count rate, in theory, reaches zero as the dead time is extended infinitely. In practice, this occurs at activities which are well beyond the levels which are allowed for patient use.

Interrelation of Spatial Resolution and Sensitivity

The spatial resolution of a parallel-hole collimator becomes poorer as the distance between the source of radioactivity and the collimator face increases. However, the sensitivity remains approximately constant. This is because the number of gamma photons passing through a particular collimator hole decreases with the square of the distance but the number of holes through which the photons can pass increases as the square of the distance. These two effects cancel each other out, leading to the sensitivity being independent of distance. This can be seen from Fig. 5.10 where the area under the profile, which equates to the sensitivity or number of events detected, is identical in both examples.

Table 5.1 shows typical system resolution and sensitivity values of a range of collimators. Even with the collimator in contact with the patient, there is still a rapid degradation of resolution with tissue depth. This fact, together with the increase in attenuation with depth, is why it is common to take more than one view in planar radionuclide imaging.

Quality Control

To allow for the most accurate images obtainable, all gamma cameras should be subject to regular quality-control tests, ideally at least consistent with the manufacturer's recommendations.

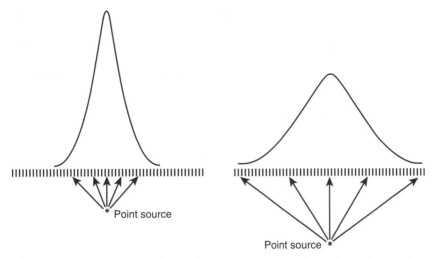

Fig. 5.10 Diagram representing the relationship between spatial resolution and sensitivity as the source of activity moves further away from the collimator face.

TABLE 5.1   Indicative Values[a] for Spatial Resolution and Sensitivity of a Typical Range of Collimators on a Gamma Camera

| Collimator Type | SPATIAL RESOLUTION FWHM (MM) | | Sensitivity (cps/MBq) for Technetium-99m |
	On Collimator Face	10 cm from Collimator	
Low-energy general purpose	5	8	160
Low-energy high resolution	4	7	110
Medium energy	6	13	185
High energy	8	15	100

[a]Different manufacturers will quote considerably different values.
FWHM, full width at half maximum.

As the spatial resolution, sensitivity, energy resolution, and count rate performance are determined by the components and construction of the detector head, these should not vary in a significant way and do not require to be checked as frequently. They should be checked when any component of the detector system, such as a PMT, has been replaced.

The uniformity, as the most variable parameter, should be checked most frequently, and ideally daily. This can be done with and/or without collimators and is tested by exposing the detector to a uniform flux of gamma photons. A point source at a distance can be used if the detector is tested without the collimators, otherwise a uniformly distributed source of a suitable radionuclide, large enough to encompass the entire detector, should be used. Fillable Perspex phantoms to which water containing $^{99}Tc^m$ can be added are available, but these can be prohibitively heavy with the large size of modern detector heads. Alternatives are uniform sources of cobalt-57 which are available commercially to fit most manufacturer's detector heads. Cobalt-57 is chosen as the 120-keV photopeak energy is close to that of technetium-99m, so the performance is similar, and the 9-month half-life allows a reasonable lifespan before the source needs to be replaced.

The uniformity is assessed using performance indices which look at variations in the count response across the entire field of view and the largest local fluctuations. These should be compared daily with the tolerances quoted by the manufacturer before the camera is used clinically. Trend analysis looking at variation of these parameters over time is also a useful tool for early identification of drift in the system performance.

PRACTICAL GAMMA CAMERA IMAGING

The most common type of imaging used in nuclear medicine is planar imaging which gives a 2D image of the 3D distribution of radioactivity within the body. There are three main categories of methods of acquiring planar images which are:
- Static imaging
- Dynamic imaging
- Gated imaging

Further detail will now be provided for some of these methods described above.

Static Imaging

Static imaging is used where the distribution of a radiopharmaceutical within the patient is changing very slowly with time and can be regarded as effectively stable for the duration of the image acquisition. Whole-body imaging, which will be described more fully later, is a form of static imaging which can be used to image an area larger than the field of view of the gamma camera.

In general, the duration of the delay between injection and the commencement of static imaging depends upon the study and the behaviour of the radiopharmaceutical. For example, dimercaptosuccinic acid (DMSA) images are acquired around 3 h after injection, whereas images of the thyroid may be acquired 15 min after injection.

Static images provide information about the target organ size, shape, and position within the body and in relation to other structures. They can also demonstrate regions of increased and/or decreased radiopharmaceutical uptake. They generally require limited processing, such as optimising image display (choice of colour scale, filtering windowing) and region of interest (ROI) analysis, as will be described later.

Whole-Body Imaging

Whole-body images are acquired in a continuous mode where the patient couch travels at a constant speed between the opposed detector heads. This allows coverage of the whole patient body in a reasonable timescale. The rate at which the couch progresses during the scan generally ranges from 6–20 cm/min. The main advantages of the technique are speed, in that it is faster than acquiring multiple static views to cover the same area, and the guarantee that no areas will be missed. The main disadvantage of whole-body scanning is that there is a theoretical loss of resolution. However, this can be minimised if the scan rate of the couch chosen correctly. Modern cameras use autocontouring systems to ensure that the detector heads are always as close as possible to the patient and to avoid collisions between the patient and the detectors. These generally use an array of LEDs on one side of the detector head with a matching array of photodetectors on the opposite side. The light beams created can be used to detect the outline of the patient and the detector set to stay at a fixed distance from this.

Dynamic Imaging

This is used where the radioactivity within the area of interest is changing rapidly with time. Multiple short-duration images, or frames, are acquired consecutively, often starting at the time of injection of the radiopharmaceutical.

In general, a series of image frames are acquired while the patient remains stationary. The length of individual frames varies from 0.1 s to >300 s depending on the study. Multiple different frame times may be used within the same study. The number and length of frames will be chosen to produce the optimal images of the changing distribution. Short frames are required when the radioactive distribution is changing most rapidly, or when the highest amount of radiopharmaceutical is present in the organ of interest, with longer frames used once the rate of change has slowed. Frame lengths are often chosen such that the total counts acquired in each frame are essentially constant during the acquisition.

Static images can be created by grouping frames together into summed images at timepoints through the acquisition. This removes the need to acquire additional static views and does not disrupt the acquisition of the dynamic data. Image processing is often required to produce useful outputs from dynamic imaging, and this can include background subtraction, ROI analysis, and generation of time activity curves (TACs).

Gated Imaging

Gated imaging is used to image organs with regular physiological motion from which a trigger signal can be obtained. The most important example is cardiac gating where the electrocardiography (ECG) signal can be used to obtain a suitable trigger.

In cardiac gated imaging, the image acquisition is triggered by the R wave of the patient's ECG. Images are acquired into a fixed number of frames for a set time per frame, so that a complete cardiac cycle fills all frames available. When the next R wave is received, information from the first portion of the cardiac cycle is added to that of the previous cycle, etc. This is repeated until a total of typically 5 million counts have been acquired.

The number of frames acquired is typically 8 or 16 for myocardial perfusion imaging and 16, 24, or 32 for radionuclide ventriculography for assessment of the left ventricular ejection fraction. The higher the number of frames, the higher the temporal resolution which can be obtained, but the data is noisier due to reduced counts in each frame.

Imaging Parameters

During routine imaging, the operator can make several choices in image acquisition, display, and processing which will affect the appearance of the image. These include:

Acquisition: **Image Processing:**
Collimator   Image filtering
Number of counts   Regions of interest
Matrix   Geometric mean
Views (orientation)   TACs
Camera-patient distance   Parametric images
Zoom
Image Display:
Look-up tables
Contrast enhancement
Display size
Collimator

Parallel-hole collimators are used for most planar imaging with typically LEGP or LEHR collimators being used. In the choice of collimator, there is always an inherent compromise between spatial resolution and sensitivity. High-resolution collimators achieve better spatial resolution images at the expense of low count rates and hence longer imaging times. High-sensitivity collimators allow a higher count rate but yield lower-resolution images and in practice are only sparingly used.

In practice, high-resolution collimators are used where small structures need to be resolved, like in bone scans. General-purpose collimators are used in dynamic images where count rate is more important than anatomical detail, like in renal imaging.

Image Counts

A high image-count density is required to achieve a high signal-to-noise ratio and hence better image quality. The count density can be increased by:

Increasing imaging time: This is limited by the need to avoid patient motion and the logistics of timing patients throughout the working day

Increasing the amount of administered radioactivity: This is limited by the legal requirement to ensure that doses are kept as low as reasonably practicable and the diagnostic reference levels (DRLs) set locally and nationally

Ensuring acceptable gamma camera sensitivity: The sensitivity of the camera should be checked periodically as part of the routine quality-control programme

Image Matrix

The pixel size sets a limit on image spatial resolution and at least two pixels per FWHM are needed to avoid loss of detail in the acquired images. Given that FWHM values are comparatively large in radionuclide imaging, this can be achieved with a relatively coarse pixel matrix.

The typical image matrices used are 64×64, 128×128, 256×256, and 512×512. Normally, images are acquired, stored, and displayed with the same matrix. The choice of matrix alters the size of the pixels as the camera's field of view is fixed. Thus, for a 540×400 mm field of view, the pixel size for 128×128 is 4.2 mm and 8.4 mm for 64×64.

At low matrix sizes, the images will appear 'coarser', so a larger matrix size should be chosen for high-quality imaging. Typically, 256×256 or 512×512 is suitable for static imaging. For dynamic imaging, 128×128 is often used, and 64×64 is the general choice for gated cardiac images.

Distance

The gamma camera should be as close as possible to the patient during imaging to optimise spatial resolution. Reducing the air gap between the patient and the camera improves spatial resolution. As discussed, autocontouring can be used to achieve this in whole-body imaging.

Zoom

It may be necessary to make an image larger by acquiring with a zoom, especially in paediatric imaging such as DMSA renal scans where the kidneys may only be a few centimetres in size. With a zoom of 2, the pixel size is halved. Reducing the pixel size by a factor of N reduces the counts per pixel by a factor of N^2, which decreases the signal-to-noise ratio, leading to another compromise between resolution and image quality.

Image Display

Images are generally displayed using a matrix in which different count values are displayed as different intensities, or colours. The relationship between pixel count and brightness/colour is defined in a look-up table. Most display screens are 8-bit, so the table has 256 (2^8) different intensities. It is generally best to avoid colour scales with discrete steps in colour between slightly differing intensities, such as those in rainbow colour scales, as these can cause difficulties with visual perception for the observer. Continuous colour scales such as hot-body or thermal options are better as they have no discrete steps and change gradually with intensity.

The image display should use a linear colour scale as non-linear displays offer too much scope for the observer to 'create' apparent abnormalities. Similarly, displays which use a 'gamma' parameter to alter the display response should be avoided or the gamma parameter should be fixed to disable user intervention to ensure consistency amongst different observers.

Windowing

As with most radiological images, the contrast in the image can be enhanced by windowing. Depending on the upper and lower window limits chosen, pixels containing high counts may be saturated or pixels containing low counts may be zeroed.

Display Size

The display screen is a large pixel array often with a few thousand pixels in each dimension on modern digital monitors. This allows display of a single image acquired in a large matrix or several images acquired with smaller matrices, allowing simultaneous display of several frames of a dynamic study or different views of the same organ. Images acquired with a smaller matrix can be displayed in the full display size by using image interpolation. This computes the contents of the additional pixels in the matrix by averaging the values of adjacent pixels in the original image.

Quality control of digital display systems is now of major importance due to the use of digital PACS for image reporting. The AAPM (American Association of Physicists in Medicine) Task Group 18[1] report is a useful resource for this purpose and includes digital test patterns for consistent quality control.

Filtering

Image filtering involves alteration of the image-count density values to achieve a specific aim, usually to smooth or enhance edges in the image. This is generally carried out by means of the mathematical technique of convolution, using a two-dimensional matrix, f, referred to as the kernel or mask.

The image is convolved with f to give the filtered image I_f.

$$I_f(x, y) = I(x, y) \times f(x, y)$$

Making the filter array larger to increase the number of pixels in each operation will increase the amount of smoothing. Changing the values of the filter to give the greatest weight to those pixels closest to the centre alters the degree of smoothing.

$$f(x, y) = \frac{1}{16} \begin{bmatrix} 1 & 2 & 1 \\ 2 & 4 & 2 \\ 1 & 2 & 1 \end{bmatrix}$$

This is a typical 9-point smoothing filter used for planar images. The factor 1/16 ensures that the mean count density in the filtered image is the same as in the original image. Smoothing filters preferentially exclude high spatial frequencies whereas edge-detection (or sharpening) filters preferentially exclude low spatial frequencies. If sharpening is required, then some kernel values will be negative.

$$f(x, y) = \begin{bmatrix} 0 & 1 & 0 \\ 1 & -4 & 1 \\ 0 & 1 & 0 \end{bmatrix}$$

More complicated and hence computationally intensive filters are applied in the frequency domain. Convolution in the spatial domain is equivalent to multiplication in the frequency domain. Convolution is thus done by multiplying the Fourier transforms of the image and filter which has the advantage of requiring less computational power than direct convolution.

The fine spatial detail in an image has the highest spatial frequencies, but this is also the frequency range predominated by image noise. Therefore, a compromise is again required as 'low-pass' filtering to exclude image noise will also remove some of the fine detail from the image. It is often the case then that observers are presented with the original raw images as well as the filtered images to allow them to make a full assessment of all aspects of the data.

Regions of Interest

ROI analysis is used to generate count statistics in a defined region of either a static or dynamic image. The area may be drawn manually by the user or automatically by the processing system using edge-detection software.

Anterior and posterior images with ROIs around a specific organ may be used to calculate the geometric mean counts in the organ. This gives some correction for depth for organs which may lie at different depths in the body, the most useful example being the kidneys.

$$\text{Geometric mean} = \sqrt{\text{anterior cts} \times \text{posterior cts}}$$

Thus, in DMSA static renal imaging, the background-corrected geometric means for each kidney are used in the calculation of relative function of the kidneys.

Time Activity Curves

ROIs defined on dynamic studies can be used to generate TACs, where points on the curve represent the number of counts within the ROI in each frame of the study. Parameters can be derived, such as the area under the curve, the curve slope, and the time to reach a peak. Processing software can carry out further manipulations such as curve fitting and extrapolation.

Parametric Imaging

TACs only demonstrate the behaviour of the radiopharmaceutical averaged within the entire ROI. Parametric images are generated by deriving a parameter from TACs for each pixel and displaying this in an image form by replacing the counts in a pixel by this parameter.

The most common example is probably the calculation of the phase and amplitude parameters for pixels within the left ventricle in radionuclide ventriculography. A sinusoidal curve is fitted to the cardiac-cycle TAC and Fourier analysis is used to find the magnitude of contraction and the time at which the maximum emptying occurs

These parameters are used to generate the amplitude and phase images of the heart, shown in Fig. 5.11. Regional wall-motion abnormalities may be seen on both images at the apex of the heart due to an aneurysmal region.

IMAGE QUALITY

Image Contrast

Contrast in a nuclear medicine image is largely determined by the differential uptake of the radiopharmaceutical in a lesion and surrounding healthy tissue. Thus, it depends primarily on physiological function rather than physical factors.

If the lesion and healthy tissue have activities A_L and A_T, respectively, the subject contrast C_S may be defined as

$$C_S = \frac{A_L - A_T}{A_T}$$

With this definition, a 'hot' lesion shows positive contrast whereas a 'cold' lesion, or photopenic defect,

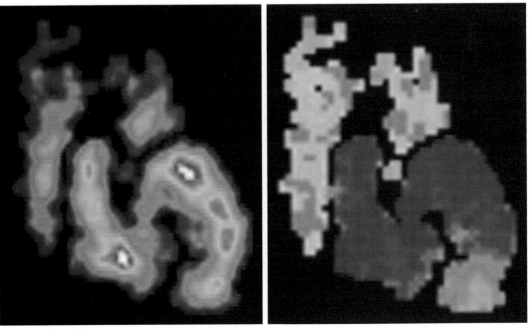

Fig. 5.11 Phase and amplitude images of the heart in a patient with an aneurysmal defect at the apex of the left ventricle.

shows negative contrast. The limit of negative contrast is -1, but there is no theoretical limit to positive contrast. For this reason, radiopharmaceuticals that produce positive contrast are generally preferred. It is also predominantly the case that human observers perform better in tasks using positive contrast.

Image contrast C_I can be defined as

$$C_I = \frac{S_L - S_T}{S_T}$$

where S_L and S_T are the count densities in the lesion and surrounding tissue respectively. The count density is generally expressed in counts per pixel. In nuclear medicine, it is generally true that C_I is almost always less than C_S due to overlying tissue.

Image Noise

In nuclear medicine, image noise may be either structured or random, sometimes referred to as coloured or white noise. Structured, or coloured, noise is due to non-random variations in count density that are superimposed upon and interfere with the objects of interest. This may arise from the physiological distribution of the radiopharmaceutical, or imaging system artefacts. Random, or white, noise is due to random variations in count density which result from the random nature of radioactive decay. It impairs the detectability of lesions, and its importance is such that radionuclide imaging is often said to be noise-limited. This is due to the low sensitivity of the gamma camera system and a limit on the radiopharmaceutical activity that may be administered to the patient.

If an image contains N counts, the random noise in that region is the standard deviation of N.

$$\sigma = \sqrt{N}$$

The signal-to-noise ratio, SNR, is defined by:

$$\mathrm{SNR} = N/\sigma = N/\sqrt{N} = \sqrt{N}$$

The relative or fractional noise, also known as the noise contrast, C_N, is given by

$$C_N = \sigma/N = \sqrt{N}/N = 1/\sqrt{N}$$

Thus, the noise contrast and the SNR are inverses of each other.

In imaging, the relative noise (noise contrast) is the more important factor, not absolute noise. Relative noise is reduced by acquiring a large number of counts. Therefore,

in planar radionuclide imaging, each image typically contains a few tens of thousands to a few million counts.

Thus, the factors that determine noise are essentially those that determine the number of counts acquired:
- Image acquisition time

  The longer the acquisition time, the lower the relative noise, but the likelihood of patient motion is increased (impairing image contrast and spatial resolution).
- Activity of radiopharmaceutical

  For a given acquisition time, relative noise decreases as the activity is increased, but at the cost of increased radiation dose.
- Sensitivity of the gamma camera system

  The greater the system sensitivity, the lower the relative noise for a given acquisition time and administered activity, as more counts will be acquired.

Contrast-to-Noise Ratio

In radionuclide imaging, even when the size of a lesion is substantially larger than the spatial resolution, random noise can impair detectability of the lesion, especially if the lesion has low contrast.

The quantity that determines lesion detectability is the contrast-to-noise ratio, CNR, which is defined as the ratio of the modulus of the image contrast to the noise contrast in the surrounding tissue.

$$\mathrm{CNR} = \frac{|C_I|}{C_N}$$

This can only be correctly defined when N is the number of counts in a region of the surrounding tissue which has the same area as the lesion.

For a lesion to be detectable, the CNR must exceed $3-5$ (depending on factors such as lesion shape, spatial resolution, viewing distance, and observer experience). This is known as the Rose criterion.

TOMOGRAPHIC IMAGING

As described earlier, planar imaging produces 2D images of a 3D radiopharmaceutical distribution with the inherent reduction in lesion contrast that this entails. Tomographic imaging enables improved contrast to be obtained by removing or reducing the effects of activity in overlying and underlying tissues, as shown in Fig. 5.12.

There are two forms of tomographic imaging in nuclear medicine which utilise both radionuclides which emit single gamma rays and positron emitters. These will be described in turn.

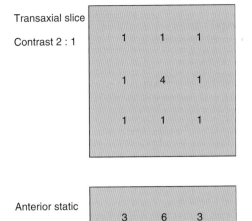

Transaxial slice

Contrast 2 : 1

Anterior static

Contrast 4 : 1

Fig. 5.12 Diagram demonstrating the improved image contrast achievable with tomographic imaging.

Single-Photon Emission Computed Tomography (SPECT)

SPECT is the technique for obtaining a 3D distribution of a single gamma ray—emitting radiopharmaceutical within the body.

Single photon — to differentiate from positron emission tomography (PET)

Emission — as the patient is the radioactive source

Computed tomography — as the acquisition and reconstruction processes are analogous to CT

Almost any radiopharmaceutical distribution can be imaged using SPECT, provided that:

- The distribution of the radiopharmaceutical does not change significantly within the duration of the image acquisition time, typically 20—40 minutes
- The acquisition time is long enough for enough gamma photons to be acquired to ensure acceptable noise levels

Important clinical applications of SPECT include:

- Cerebral blood flow
- Skeletal imaging
- Myocardial perfusion
- Neuroendocrine tumour imaging

Gamma camera systems use 2D detectors and as such are inherently multislice or volume devices. Data must be acquired from all angles around the patient before any slices can be generated, and the acquisition data, usually called projection data, is reconstructed into a series of tomographic images using computational reconstruction techniques.

The most common SPECT systems are the dual-headed arrangements as shown earlier in Fig. 5.5. The detector heads can generally be positioned opposing each other (180° mode) or at right angles to one another (90° mode). Some systems allow positioning at further intermediate angles (for example, 76°) for specific applications or collimator configurations.

Quality Control for SPECT

The gamma camera performance requirements for SPECT are more stringent than for planar imaging as the design and performance of the detectors, collimators, gantry, and patient table can have a significant impact on SPECT image quality.

Poor performance of any aspect of the SPECT system will result in very similar image artefacts within the final reconstructed SPECT slices. These artefacts are often circular in nature, can be either 'hot' or 'cold', and are generally referred to as 'ring' artefacts.

Detector Energy Resolution

The energy resolution of modern detectors is <10% which is more than adequate for performing SPECT. The lower the energy resolution, the better the system at minimising scatter effects and the better the image contrast obtained.

Detector Uniformity

SPECT images are created from different views of the same radiopharmaceutical distribution, and so the detector response should ideally be the same at all acquisition angles. However, PMTs are susceptible to minute fluctuations in the Earth's magnetic field as the detectors rotate and this can cause non-uniform response. The SPECT uniformity of the system should be checked at least monthly and the calculated performance indices should be within tolerance at all angles.

Gantry Centre of Rotation

Modern gantries provide accurate, stable rotation and alignment of the camera heads as they rotate around the patient. The mechanical rotation of the camera heads should be perfectly circular, and the rotational centre must accurately align with the centre of data reconstruction. If the two do not intersect, a centre of rotation (COR) offset is defined by the separation between them. The COR is measured from a series of images of a small point source taken from multiple angles around the source. The source should be in the centre of the field of view, offset by ~15 cm from the axis of rotation, and a SPECT acquisition obtained such that there are sufficient counts in each projection to accurate locate the centre of the source.

The X and Y coordinates of the point source are plotted against image angle and compared to an ideal sine wave. The offsets between the data and the ideal line are stored for X and Y as a function of the acquisition angle and are used to shift all SPECT projection data by the required X and Y values, prior to image reconstruction.

Gantry Detector Alignment

The face of the camera heads must be aligned parallel to the mechanical axis of rotation to minimise distortions in the reconstructed images. This is particularly important in systems with variable head configurations and will generally be checked by the engineers as part of the routine maintenance programme.

Collimator

To obtain optimal SPECT images, the collimator holes should be as parallel as possible, and the hole size and septal thickness should be as uniform as possible. Therefore, cast collimators are much preferred for SPECT as they are more uniform than foil collimators, although significantly more expensive.

As a safety feature, pressure-sensitive touchpads are fitted to the front of the collimators to detect any contact between the collimators and the patient. If these are activated, all gantry motion will be immediately disabled, or, in some systems, the detector heads will immediately move away to their maximum radius position.

In SPECT, the detector-to-patient distance should always be minimised to maximise the resolution obtained. This is known as 'body contouring' and is achieved by the same autocontouring devices used for whole-body imaging.

Patient Table

The design and construction of the patient table is important for the safety and comfort of the patient during SPECT acquisition. This is important as comfortable patients keep still, thus minimising movement artefacts in the final images.

Qualitative Assessment of Performance

As well as quantitative assessment, the overall tomographic performance of the system can be visually assessed from SPECT images acquired using a Jaszczak test object. This is a cylindrical tank containing various sized Perspex rods and spheres which span a range around that which is expected to be resolvable in the images. These assessments are of overall system performance and therefore identifying which factor is degrading performance can take considerable investigation.

Acquisition Parameters

The choice of parameters for the acquisition of projection data depends on several factors. As most of these factors are interdependent, the final choice may involve compromises. However, the ability of the patient to keep still is the overriding factor in determining final image quality.

Acquisition Matrix

The chosen matrix size determines the spatial sampling (maximum resolution), counts per pixel (image noise), and minimum slice thickness of the SPECT data. Large matrices (and hence small pixel size) produce the best resolution and thinnest slices but at the expense of high image noise. If possible, a 128×128 matrix should be used to maximise image resolution, but this will depend on the count density in the organ of interest. Image post-processing can offset the impact of image noise to some extent by increasing the slice thickness, using smoother filters, or displaying the data in a lower-resolution (e.g., 64×64) matrix, or a combination of these.

Projection Views

Projection Time. The acquisition time per projection is typically 20–40 s for most SPECT studies. This time depends upon the administered activity, and hence count density in the organ of interest, choice of collimator, and the specific uptake within the patient themselves. Some methods are now available to accelerate frame times to 5–10 s.

Rotation. The detector heads can be rotated in either continuous or 'step-and-shoot' mode. In continuous mode, the detector rotates at a constant speed and data is acquired throughout the rotation. The step-and-shoot mode moves the camera head to each discrete projection angle and then stops for the requisite acquisition time before moving to the next angle. This is generally considered preferable as the camera is stationary during the acquisition, but it takes longer to acquire the data which increases the risk of patient movement.

Angular Step. The angular sampling used should be similar to spatial sampling. This means that the step angle should be approximately the rotation length divided by the number of reconstructed slices which derives from the matrix size. Therefore, 3° steps should be used for a 128×128 matrix and a 360° rotation.

Angular Range. Generally, projection data should be acquired over 360° with the heads opposed for all SPECT scans, except myocardial perfusion imaging. The use of 360° acquisition allows averaging of projections which can reduce artefacts and geometrical distortion. The exception in cardiac imaging is due to the very anterior location of the heart within the chest. The use of 360° acquisition actually degrades the quality in cardiac imaging in comparison to a 180° angular range due to the amount of scatter present in the projections from the posterior of the patient. However, this may not be the case if a CT scan is to be used for correction of attenuation in cardiac imaging and a full 360° acquisition is required.

Collimator

The collimator choice is a compromise decision for the operator between improving resolution or sensitivity. As lower sensitivity can be overcome by increasing the acquisition time but resolution cannot be restored, a high-resolution collimator should be used wherever possible. This also reduces image distortion during the reconstruction process as these collimators give better preservation of resolution with distance from the collimator. This can also be improved by use of body-contoured orbits which ensure that the patient-collimator distance is minimised.

Patient Factors

There are several patient-related factors which can affect overall image quality and be the cause of artefacts in SPECT.

Motion

Patients must keep as still as possible during acquisition to minimise artefacts. Any motion of greater than the dimension of 2 pixels may introduce artefacts into the reconstructed images. For example, for a 64 × 64 matrix, movement of more than ~16 mm is necessary before an artefact may be seen.

Injection Site

Any injection site should be kept out of the field of view during acquisition to avoid the possibility of introducing artefacts into the reconstructed images.

Arm Position

As has been mentioned previously, resolution is improved by minimising the distance between the patient and the detector. Therefore, for SPECT of the chest or heart, the patient's arms should be kept above their heads if possible.

However, some patients may be unable to tolerate this. Positioning the arms out of the field of view also avoids possible truncation artefacts.

Image Reconstruction
Filtered Back Projection

The original back-projection techniques used for SPECT image reconstruction originated in radioastronomy prior to the Second World War and are based on the mathematical techniques of convolution and Fourier transformation.

The process can be divided into three separate stages:
- Creation of 1D profiles from each projection angle
- Filtering of these profiles
- 'Back projection' of the filtered profiles

This is all done in frequency space using convolution and Fourier transforms to optimise speed and minimise computational requirements.

Projection Profiles. As the camera rotates around the patient, a 1D profile of the radionuclide distribution is taken.

Back Projection. This is the mathematical process which creates an image from the acquired profile values. The profile value at each point is back-projected across the new image to fill each pixel with the profile value along the line of the angle of the profile. This is then repeated for all profiles (angles) to build up the final image. However, the image created is noisy and poor quality with a noticeable 'star' artefact in the image background, as shown in Fig. 5.13.

Filtering. The noise and star effects in the background can be reduced by filtering the profiles. The filter usually performs some form of smoothing to reduce the influence of the higher spatial frequencies. The filter function used often has 'negative tails' as this helps to minimise background effects.

Filtered Back Projection. Repeating the back-projection process with filtered profile data results in an image with reduced noise and removal of the 'star' artefact. The

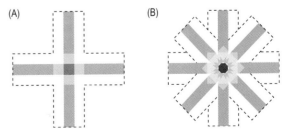

Fig. 5.13 Diagram of the back-projection process demonstrating the 'star' artefact.

resultant image appears closer to the true distribution of the radionuclide but with some degree of blurring, which is an inherent part of the back-projection process.

Reconstruction Filters. The filter kernel chosen for the profiles is always a compromise between reducing the noise in the final image and the resolution achievable. The degree of smoothing achieved is defined by the cut-off, or critical frequency, of the filter which determines the maximum spatial frequency present in the reconstructed image. On most systems, several different filters are available, the most common of which include the Butterworth & Hanning kernels.

Iterative Reconstruction

Filtered back projection (FBP) is simple computationally and fast to implement but it does not produce an exact mathematical solution. The alternative is to use an iterative reconstruction (IR) technique as these do converge to an optimal solution, but they are computationally complex. With the increasing computer power available in the last decade or so, the use of IR techniques has become the preferred option.

One major difference of IR techniques is that they require an *a priori* estimate of the distribution of the radionuclide. However, in nuclear medicine, this can often just be an ellipse filled with a uniform value, although faster convergence can be achieved with more realistic starting estimates.

This initial estimate is forward-projected to produce an estimated projection set which is compared with the original projection data. A difference image between these is then created and back-projected. This is then used as the starting estimate for the next iteration of the process. This process is repeated iteratively until the differences, calculated by one of a range of mathematical methods, are minimised. A schematic of this process can be seen in Fig. 5.14. An important advantage for nuclear medicine is

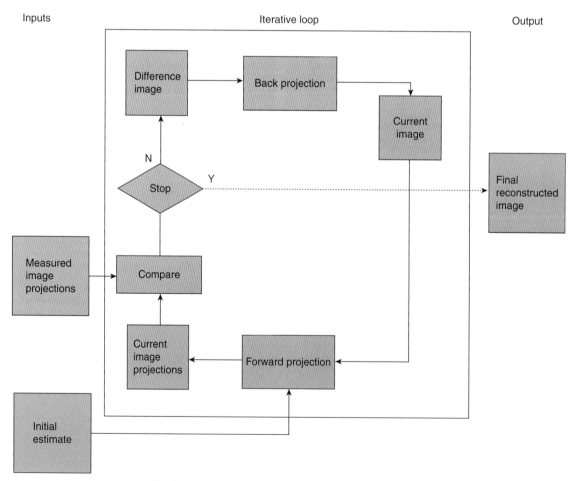

Fig. 5.14 Diagram of the iterative reconstruction process.

that IR methods can incorporate corrections for both attenuation and scatter during the iterative loop.

Most SPECT data is now reconstructed using iterative methods as there are accelerated algorithms now available which make reconstruction times clinically acceptable. The most common of these is the ordered subsets expectation maximisation (OSEM) algorithm in which adjacent groups of projections, which are inherently similar, are grouped together in subsets then reconstructed. The reconstruction is accelerated by a factor proportional to the number of subsets.

Attenuation

Attenuation of the gamma radiation within the patient is a significant problem in SPECT, particularly if it is non-uniform. This is most apparent when imaging the heart within the chest where there are differing attenuation properties from bone, air, soft tissue, and blood.

The effects of attenuation can be corrected for by using analytical techniques or by direct measurement.

Analytical

If attenuation can be assumed to be uniform within the object, then analytical techniques can be used to correct for the effects of attenuation. The most common of these is the Chang method, which assumes that attenuation varies exponentially with distance and that the patient outline can be accurately defined. The pixel counts within the image are thus scaled according to the distance from the camera. However, the only region of the body where these assumptions can be found with any degree of certainty is in the head, where the attenuation values of grey and white brain matter and cerebrospinal fluid are approximately equal.

Direct Measurement

Direct measurements of the attenuation coefficients within the body can be obtained using external transmission sources (e.g., using a radionuclide such as gadolinium-153) or a CT system. Both involve additional radiation dose to the patient, but this is generally less for CT systems due to the shorter exposure times required. External radionuclide sources are also subject to decay and require replacement on a regular basis which can add considerably to overall costs. If a CT system is used, the dataset obtained is an attenuation map of the patient which can be incorporated into the OSEM algorithm.

Display — Projection Data

As a quality check, the projection data from a patient should be visually assessed prior to reconstruction to identify potential issues which may lead to artefacts in the final data.

A rotating cine view of the projection data can be used to check for:
- Possible patient motion
- Incomplete datasets due to truncation
- Interference from injection site
- Possible attenuation arising from metal objects, arms, breasts, etc.

The projection data can also be displayed and assessed as a sinogram, where pixel values from a single projection are summed and stacked by angle. Discontinuities or missing slices within the sinogram can indicate similar issues to those listed above but a greater degree of operator familiarity is required to adequately assess these.

Display — 3D

As would be expected, SPECT data can be best viewed in 3D where the entire dataset is visible. There are two main methods used for creating 3D data for display: surface rendering (SR) or maximum intensity projection (MIP) algorithms. In practice, SR is of little use in nuclear medicine due to the functional nature of the data as the signals from deeper within the patient tend to be obscured. In MIP, the pixel intensity in the 3D object is the maximum intensity along the projection line from the pixel to the viewing plane. This works best when the object of interest in the image dataset is the brightest, which is generally the case in nuclear medicine images.

Hybrid Imaging

One of the most important advancements in nuclear medicine in recent years has been the development of hybrid imaging systems, where CT capability has become available on dual-head systems. The CT function is not used for planar imaging but can be combined with SPECT data to produce 'fused' SPECT/CT datasets. These allow fusion of SPECT (functional) and CT (anatomical) images which can greatly enhance the ability of the person reporting the data to localise pathology. CT can also be used to perform accurate attenuation correction of the SPECT images, especially when IR algorithms are used.

SPECT/CT imaging is now considered to be the standard of care for many nuclear medicine imaging examinations. This is especially true of examinations which produce lesions with increased uptake within soft tissue where there are few anatomical landmarks visible.

These hybrid systems generally employ a fan-beam X-ray source and detector array mounted on the gantry. A full range of CT capabilities are now available on commercial SPECT/CT systems from low-dose, low-resolution systems with two slices up to 64-slice systems with full diagnostic capability. The limiting factor to the utility of these systems is that the two imaging systems are not truly co-located and cannot image the same volume of the patient simultaneously. The patient must be moved between the two imaging systems and the images acquired consecutively. This introduces the possibility of the patient moving between the two scans and introducing misregistration into the fused images.

Positron Emission Tomography

PET is a tomographic radionuclide imaging technique showing physiological function, in many respects similar to SPECT. However, PET radionuclides decay by positron emission and imaging therefore relies on the detection of the pair of collinear photons resulting from the annihilation of the positron and an electron. These photons are detected by a ring of radiation detectors which removes the need for physical collimation and greatly increases the sensitivity of the detector system. Near-simultaneous detection of the photons allows localisation of their origin to a line joining the detectors, which is called annihilation coincidence detection (ACD).

Positron Annihilation and Range

As described earlier in Chapter 1, the positron e^+ is the antiparticle of the electron and once emitted will annihilate with a free electron as soon as possible, producing two collinear 511-keV photons. In tissue, positrons lose most of their energy through collisions with bound electrons, causing excitations and ionisations which contribute most of the radiation dose to the patient in PET. The positrons lose energy and are deflected at each collision, and so their paths are tortuous and unpredictable. Therefore, the range of the positron in tissue is also variable. The range is the distance between the point of emission and the point of annihilation and is typically of the order of a few millimetres for most PET radionuclides. This introduces a fundamental limit to the spatial resolution of a PET imaging system as it can never be less than the positron range.

PET Radionuclides

The most widely used radionuclide in PET imaging is fluorine-18, which accounts for at least 85% of use in the UK. It is cyclotron-produced and the half-life of 109 min makes remote production and transport to the imaging site feasible. This is unlike most other common positron emitters which have shorter half-lives of, at most, a few

TABLE 5.2   Common Positron Emission Tomography Radionuclides

Radionuclide	Half-life (min)	Source
Carbon-11	20.4	Cyclotron
Fluorine-18	109.8	Cyclotron
Gallium-68	68.3	Generator or cyclotron
Rubidium-82	1.3	Generator

tens of minutes, making on site production necessary. Table 5.2 shows several of the most common PET radionuclides currently in use with their physical parameters.

The cyclotron targets used in PET radionuclide production are generally gaseous or aqueous, but can be solid, and these are irradiated mainly with protons. Deuterons, ^2H, or helium nuclei, ^3He or ^4He, can also be used for target bombardment but these require higher power requirements due to their greater mass and may be beyond the capability of some systems.

PET Radiopharmaceuticals

As stated previously, the most common PET radiopharmaceutical is ^{18}F-fluorodeoxyglucose (**FDG**) due to its utility in oncology. It is relatively easy to synthesise and can be produced with a high radiochemical yield, generally >90%. FDG follows a similar metabolic pathway to glucose *in vivo*, both undergoing phosphorylation in the cell, but it remains trapped within the cells and does not undergo further metabolism due to the negative charge on the phosphate group attached to the phosphorylated FDG. There are several other radiopharmaceuticals useful for oncology imaging, including ^{11}C methionine for imaging of protein synthesis, which can be disrupted in several pathologies.

In addition to oncology, PET also has applications in cardiology, neurology, and infection imaging. Oxygen-15 (^{15}O) in the form of gaseous oxygen or labelled water may be used to monitor blood flow, which has uses in several pathologies and research applications.

Myocardial perfusion may be imaged with nitrogen-13 (^{13}N) ammonia or more commonly ionic rubidium-82 (^{82}Rb) which is now available commercially via a strontium-82 ($^{82}Sr/^{82}Rb$) generator.

Due to their short half-lives and the high-energy photons produced, most PET synthesis is automated using computer-controlled modules. There are several commercial sources for these, and the chemicals and reagents required to complete the synthesis are contained in cartridges which easily slot into the modules. These are generally located within 'hot cells' which are heavily shielded, with up to 15 cm of lead shielding, to maintain a safe working environment. Like all other radiopharmaceutical production, PET facilities come under the Good Manufacturing Practice regulations and are subject to Medicine and Healthcare products Regulation Agency inspection.

PET Gantry Design

Similar to gamma cameras, the annihilation gamma radiation is generally detected by scintillation crystals in a PET system. The crystals are arranged in blocks laid in a ring around the gantry with the patient bore in the centre typically having a diameter of around 70 cm. The axial field of view of the scanner is determined by the width of the ring of crystals, typically around ~15 cm. This length determines how much of the patient can be imaged at any given time and is often known as a bed or couch position. The couch moves axially, and it takes about 5–7 couch positions to cover the required field of view of the patient. This is often from the base of the brain to mid-thigh as most lesions expected to be seen in oncology imaging occur within these locations. Scanners with larger fields of view are now commercially available with the ability to scan more than 30 cm of the patient in a single bed position. However, these are more expensive due to the costs of the increased crystals required.

PET Scintillation Crystals

The requirements for a PET scintillator material are as follows:
- High attenuation properties at 511 keV (i.e., high density and effective atomic number)
- High ratio of photoelectric to Compton scatter interactions
- High light output to produce good energy resolution

- Short scintillation light decay time to allow high count rates to be handled

Table 5.3 lists the properties of several the scintillator materials used in PET systems. Sodium iodide, as used in gamma cameras, is not useful for PET due to its low attenuation at 511 keV and its long light decay which causes overlap of successive pulses at high count rates. Bismuth germinate (BGO) was the most common PET crystal for many years due to its high attenuation and relatively low cost, but it also had long light decay, limiting the count rates which were attainable. Recently, lutetium oxyorthosilicate (LSO) and similar variants such as LYSO (LSO doped with yttrium) were developed, which have high attenuation and short light decay, which mean they are now the crystals of choice.

Detector Blocks

To simplify construction and facilitate ease of maintenance, the crystals in the detector ring are organised into blocks known as detector blocks. These can then be grouped into modules of typically 8 detector blocks, which can be easily replaced when faulty. Typically, the light in each block is spread across 4 PMTs and different amounts of light reach each PMT depending on the event position within the block.

The crystal in each block is generally subdivided into an array of detector elements by cutting partial slits of varying depths. The cuts are deepest at the edges, so that the light passes down a single crystal element, and shallowest in the centre, so that the light is shared between several crystal elements. The pattern of the light sharing across the block PMTs is used to determine the event position. Each crystal element is a few square millimetres but each block of crystal is several centimetres deep. Typical modern systems will have upwards of 10,000 crystals within the detector field of view, arranged in rings. There are generally a few tens of crystals along the axial plane, often 24 crystals, and this determines the number of reconstructed slices within the field of view of each bed

TABLE 5.3	Physical Properties of Common Positron Emission Tomography Scintillator Materials			
Scintillator Material	Density (g/cm^3)	Effective Atomic Number	Relative Light Output (%)	Light Decay Time (ns)
Sodium iodide	3.7	51	100	230
Bismuth germanate	7.1	75	15	300
Lutetium oxyorthosilicate	7.4	71	75	40
Barium fluoride	4.9	45	80	0.8

position. If there are 24 crystals axially, then there are 24 direct planes for coincidence interactions between the opposite sides of each ring, plus 23 indirect planes for interactions between adjacent rings. This example gives a total for 47 reconstructed slices in each bed position.

Coincidence Detection

The electronic collimation of ACD determines the direction of travel of the photons without the need for physical collimation. If the two annihilation photons are detected simultaneously by two detectors in opposite parts of the ring, then the point of origin of the positron annihilation lies along a line joining the detector elements. The time of arrival of each photon can be recorded to a precision of ~2 ns. The two photon signals are considered coincident when they arrive within a coincidence timing window of around 10 ns. This timing window can generally be adjusted by the user within a typical range of about 6–12 ns. A longer window increases sensitivity but also increases the probability of including unwanted events due to random coincidences.

Image Formation

The imaginary line joining the two crystal elements which have detected the coincident photons is known as the line of response (LoR). Each line is stored in memory prior to reconstruction of the images. LoRs can be generated by true, scatter, or random coincidences as shown in Fig. 5.15.

- True coincidences are where the two annihilation photons are detected without interaction and the correct LoR is defined.
- Scatter coincidences are where one or both photons have undergone Compton interactions prior to detection and an erroneous LoR is defined.

- Random coincidences are where two photons from separate annihilation reactions are detected within the coincidence window and accepted as a coincident pair. Again, an erroneous LoR is defined.

The data from each bed position is essentially stored as a separate acquisition before reconstruction. However, the sensitivity of the system varies markedly in the axial direction from a peak at the centre of the field of view, falling off almost to zero at the edges. Therefore, the data from adjacent fields of view must be overlapped to ensure that the variations in sensitivity are minimised. This generally means that the couch is not moved by the full distance of the axial field of view between each acquisition, allowing the overlap to be created. The proportion of overlap can be up to 50% and is generally also under user control to allow the optimal choice of trade-off between axial sensitivity and acquisition time.

Similar to SPECT, the data acquisition may be gated to a physiological trigger. This is generally the cardiac ECG, but respiratory gating is also used in PET to attempt to clarify the exact position of small lesions in the lower lungs and liver. This is required as the CT acquisition takes only a few seconds to cover the chest and is generally within a single breathing cycle, whereas the PET acquisition will take place over several minutes and the lesion position will be averaged over multiple breathing cycles.

It should also be noted that in PET, unlike SPECT, all possible projections of data are acquired simultaneously.

Time of Flight

This is a method of improving spatial resolution by narrowing down the location of the original positron annihilation to a specific region of the LoR. This is done by measuring the time difference Δt between the annihilation photons reaching the opposed detectors.

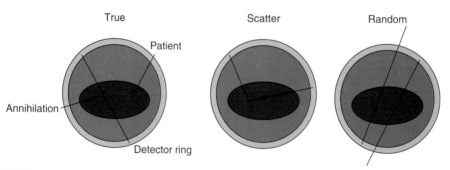

Fig. 5.15 Diagram showing the lines of response being detected when the PET scanner is imaging true, scatter, and random coincidences.

The exact location of the annihilation is then given by:

$$\Delta d = (\Delta t \times c)/2$$

where Δd is the diameter of the sphere of space to which the annihilation event can be localised, and c is the speed of light.

Localising the annihilation to a region with 1-cm resolution (diameter) requires a timing resolution of 67 ps which is beyond the capability of the light decay produced by LSO. Very fast light decay is needed, and barium fluoride (BaF_2) is the only crystal material capable of meeting this. However, its other properties are poor, and it is therefore only found in specialist research systems. With LSO, a spatial localisation of around 10 cm can be achieved which is still a considerable step forward from the generation of scanner systems with BGO crystals.

Data Correction — Scatter and Random Coincidences

As we have seen, scatter and random coincidences generate erroneous LoRs which reduce image contrast and degrade resolution. Scatter correction can be done using *a priori* estimates from phantom studies and by pulse height analysis and photopeak windowing, similar to a gamma camera. However, the energy resolution of LSO is poorer than sodium iodide and therefore a wider photopeak window is generally required in PET.

Random correction is typically done using a method of delay-line coincidences. The digital signal from the detectors is split into two and one path is delayed by an amount of time greater than the coincidence timing window set for the acquisition. Coincidences are then detected between the two paths which can be assured to be truly random. This is then subtracted from the detected signal prior to reconstruction. However, it should be noted that the events being subtracted are not the actual random coincidences but just a fraction of the signal, which is proportionate to the rate of random coincidences, and will contain true random and scatter events.

Data Correction — Other Corrections

There are a few other corrections which must be made to the data prior to reconstruction. These will now be considered in turn:

Normalisation: As has been mentioned, a typical scanner has ~15,000 detector elements, each with different efficiencies. The correction for these differing efficiencies is called normalisation and is done by exposing all detectors to a uniform photon flux, generally from an internal germanium-68 (^{68}Ge) pin source which rotates around the outer edge of the scanner bore, or a cylindrical phantom containing a uniform distribution of ^{68}Ge.

Dead time: Dead time is the finite processing time of an individual event to be handled by the system electronics, during which subsequent events will not be processed and are lost. This can be corrected using a mathematical model of detector behaviour.

Radioactive decay: As scans are acquired over several bed positions, the total acquisition may take 30 min or so. This is a significant proportion of the physical half-life of many of the PET radionuclides and the detected counts are therefore corrected for decay.

Reconstruction

Clinical PET data is now generally reconstructed using IR with accelerated algorithms (i.e., OSEM), as these allow the inclusion of all corrections mentioned above. Several manufacturers have developed proprietary reconstruction methods using statistical methods to minimise the propagation of noise during the reconstruction process and optimise resolution.

Due to the cheaper cost of computer memory, large parallel-processing arrays are now used to accelerate hardware performance and reduce reconstruction times. The dataset for a PET reconstruction may be a thousand times larger than that for a typical SPECT reconstruction. Therefore, a typical 7-bed position PET dataset will reconstruct in ~10 min. This is acceptable as faster and lower-quality reconstructions can be available in real time to allow the patient data to be checked prior to letting the patient leave the department.

Image Quality

Contrast. Random and scatter coincidences add background to the reconstructed images, thus reducing image contrast. With random coincidences, this background is relatively uniform but it is greater towards the centre of the image for scatter coincidences. Therefore, correction before reconstruction is important for optimal contrast.

Noise. The sensitivity of the PET scanner is determined by the following factors:

- Intrinsic detection efficiency — a high intrinsic efficiency requires good stopping power and thick crystals
- Geometric detection efficiency — this is the fraction of the emitted photons that reach the detectors

- Width of the photopeak acceptance window — a wide window increases scatter coincidences but also improves sensitivity

The thicker detection crystals and lack of physical collimators mean that PET sensitivity is much greater than SPECT (by a factor of ~100) and so PET images are less noisy. The image noise is affected by the choice of reconstruction technique, but IR is generally superior to FBP.

Resolution. The spatial resolution in PET is determined by the following factors:

- The positron range in tissue
- Non-collinearity of the annihilation photons, which occurs if the positron has not lost all its energy at the time of annihilation
- The size of the crystal detector elements
- The depth of the photon interaction in the detectors

Typical values of PET spatial resolution in the image plane are around 4.5 mm at the centre and 5 mm at periphery of the detector ring. The values across the field of view in the axial plane are around 4.6 mm at the centre and 6 mm at the edges. It should be noted that these values are in air and not in tissue where resolution will be degraded but not as significantly as it is in SPECT due to the higher photon energies.

Quality Control

When all corrections are applied, there should be a linear relationship between activity in the patient and counts in the reconstructed image voxels. The scanner is calibrated to achieve this by scanning a uniform cylinder of own concentration of radioactivity for a period sufficient to obtain data with a low proportion of image noise. This is known as a well counter correction.

Each scanner should be subject to a rigorous quality-control programme with tests being carried out daily, weekly, and quarterly.

The daily tests should involve a CT air check, which acquires short CT exposures using the most common combinations of kV, mA and spot sizes, and a PET uniformity check. This checks the uniformity of the response across the detectors and crystals using a ^{68}Ge source.

The weekly tests generally involve a CT quality check which looks at the accuracy of CT Hounsfield values for common materials such as air, water, and Perspex. The high voltage gain over the PMTs and crystals should be checked using a ^{68}Ge source and any necessary adjustments made.

Some of the quarterly PET and CT checks may be carried out by a service engineer if the scanner is on a service contract but some should also be carried out by the user, including the PET crystal position check, which ensures that each crystal in the ring detects a valid photopeak, and a coincidence timing check, which assesses the consistency of the coincidence windows. The well counter check should also be carried out at least quarterly. Most manufacturers will also generally recommend a quarterly check of the alignment between the PET and CT gantries, often using a proprietary phantom. The CT scanner should also be subject to the same annual checks by the local radiation protection team like other diagnostic CT system.

Hybrid and Digital PET Imaging

All commercially available system are inherently hybrid systems as it is no longer possible to buy a PET-only detector system. However, there are now PET/magnetic resonance imaging (MRI) systems available in addition to the common PET/CT systems. These are still relatively rare due to their high capital costs (roughly double that of a PET/CT system) and a lack of clinical indications where they offer a clear advantage over PET/CT systems. The use of MRI improves soft tissue contrast but makes it more difficult to attenuation-correct the PET data as there is no clear correlation between MRI tissue signal and attenuation properties for 511-keV photons. The most likely applications are those such as neurological imaging and breast studies where soft tissue contrast is of greatest importance.

The fundamental problem with a PET/MRI system is that the PMTs in a PET detector do not function correctly in the presence of large magnetic fields. The need to solve this problem led to the development of solid-state light detection solutions and this has then driven the development of digital PET/CT systems. Unlike digital gamma camera systems where the entire detection process can be done by the CZT detectors, in digital PET systems the scintillation crystals are maintained as the stopping power of the solid-state detectors is insufficient for 511-keV photons.

The PMTs are replaced by avalanche photodiodes (APDs) which detect the light signals from the crystals and send a digital signal to the processing system. The use of these in PET/MRI systems gives them the advantage that they can be co-located within the main magnet of the MRI scanner and the system can scan the same volume of the patient simultaneously, thus removing the problems of patient movement between the scans which occur in PET/CT systems.

The problem of patient movement persists in PET/CT systems as these remain essentially two separate scanners contained within one casing. There is no real integration between the systems other than the controlled motion of the patient table and couch top. The CT system is generally at the front of the gantry and the PET detector ring at the rear. Systems are now available with fully diagnostic CT capability at 128 slices and beyond. The patient is placed on the couch and an anatomical landmark set to allow accurate imaging. The operator then uses the CT scout view to determine the field of view which is to be scanned. The patient couch top makes the movement required to acquire the CT of this volume. The entire patient table then moves a distance which exactly matches the distance between the centres of the CT and PET detector rings. The same patient couch top movement is then repeated to acquire the PET data and, if the patient has not moved, then the exact same volume of the patient will have been imaged in both modalities.

RADIATION PROTECTION AND DOSIMETRY

Unlike in radiology, the radiation dose to the patient in nuclear medicine is not determined by the time it takes to acquire the image(s). It is determined by the nature of the radiopharmaceutical, its activity, its route of administration, and the biological half-life. The energy responsible for the dose is deposited in the body through ionisations caused by Compton recoil electrons and photoelectrons from gamma interactions with tissues. There may also be contributions from beta particles, internal conversion electrons, and Auger electrons. With sufficient information, it is possible to estimate the absorbed and equivalent dose to organs and tissues and the effective dose to the whole body.

For most imaging examinations, the amount of radioactivity administered is a fixed amount equivalent to the DRL and calculation of the dose to the patient is relatively straightforward. The DRLs for nuclear medicine examinations in the UK are set by ARSAC[2] (see Ch. 2) and are determined as a balanced calculation between optimising image quality and minimising radiation dose to the patient. The activities administered to paediatric patients are scaled by bodyweight with the aim of maintaining the same image quality as is obtained in adults. The DRLs for certain examinations can be exceeded if the patients are considerably larger than the norm. This must be done with the consent of the practitioner who holds the licence for the particular examination in question.

Most nuclear medicine examinations give the patients an effective dose of less than 5 mSv, which is equivalent to around 2 years of background radiation exposure for the average person in the UK. Table 5.4 lists the effective dose for several common nuclear medicine examinations.

Obviously, any additional images required, such as SPECT acquisitions, do not add further dose to the patient as the radiopharmaceutical is only injected once and images can be obtained as frequently as required until the radionuclide has decayed to a point where imaging requires too much time. However, any CT acquisitions obtained in conjunction with SPECT imaging will add an additional dose, and this must be considered carefully when the operator is justifying the additional exposures. For example, if the patient has had a recent diagnostic CT of the area in question, then the CT acquisition may be avoided and only SPECT data acquired.

The IR(ME)R legislation[3] states that an individual dosimetry calculation should be done for all patients, and this is of greatest importance for those undergoing therapeutic administrations of beta- and alpha-emitting radionuclides. There are several software packages available to assist in the calculation of the dosimetry using imaging at fixed time points after the therapeutic administration and dose rate measurements from the patient. Many of these

TABLE 5.4 DRLs and Effective Doses for a Range of Common Nuclear Medicine Imaging Examinations and Nonimaging Measurement of GFR		
Study	**DRL (MBq)**	**Effective Dose (mSv)**
Planar bone imaging	600	2.9
SPECT bone imaging	800	3.9
MAG3 renogram	100	0.7
Myocardial perfusion imaging	800	5.5–7.2[a]
^{123}I-Ioflupane brain imaging	185	4.6
^{75}Se-SeHCAT imaging	0.4	0.3
GFR measurement	10	0.05

[a]Depends upon radiopharmaceutical and technique used.
DRL, diagnostic reference level; *GFR*, glomerular filtration rate; *MAG3*, mercapto acetyl tri glycine; *SPECT*, single-photon emission computed tomography; *SeHCAT*, selenium-75 homocholic acid taurine.

utilise the Medical Internal Radiation Dose (MIRD) methodology[4] developed by the American Society of Nuclear Medicine. This uses the concept of source organs, which are those that accumulate the injected radionuclide, and target organs, which are irradiated by the radiation from the source organs. There are several additional factors which must be considered, such as patient morphology, age, sex, medication, and diet. The potential variability in these mean that the dosimetry calculations are never exact but give a reasonable estimate of the expected dose.

Nuclear Medicine Radiation Protection

As discussed in Chapter 2, the IRR17 legislation[5] dictates the designation of the environment and the precautions and personal protective equipment (PPE) required for staff. All imaging and injecting rooms will be controlled areas due to the prevailing dose rates and risk of contamination. Ideally, departments will have segregated waiting rooms keeping patients who are awaiting injection and those who have been injected and are awaiting imaging separate. These are often referred to as 'cold' and 'hot' waiting areas. The 'hot' waiting area may be a controlled or supervised area depending on the results of local risk assessment. Access to designated areas must be controlled using swipe-card systems or similar systems, and monitoring systems must be in place to allow staff to check themselves for contamination before leaving the area.

Staff who have the potential to be exposed to the risk of contamination must be supplied with appropriate PPE. This may include a uniform, disposable aprons and gloves, eye protection, and, if required, disposable protective sleeves to protect the arms. Staff should also have appropriate personal monitoring equipment to allow accurate assessment of their equivalent and effective doses. This will include film badges for assessment of whole-body dose and thermoluminescent dosimeters for assessment of extremity dose, typically to the fingers. These can be worn as stalls over the tips of the fingers or rings worn around the base of the finger. Both can be problematic for staff involved in the delicate manipulation of unsealed sources during the drawing up of radiopharmaceuticals into syringes for injection.

PET Radiation Protection

Patients

The radiation dosimetry in PET is similar to all other nuclear medicine, as the dose to the patient is proportional to activity administered and depends on physical and physiological clearance parameters. As has been stated, most of the absorbed dose in PET is delivered by the positrons during their tissue interactions rather than the high-energy photons. These tend to penetrate through the patient's body with little interaction.

When [18]FDG is administered by intravenous injection, the whole-body effective dose is 0.02 mSv/MBq. For most clinical uses of FDG, the DRL set by ARSAC is 400 MBq, resulting in an effective dose of 8 mSv per examination. Many centres now use weight-based administration regimes where 3–4 MBq/kg is given, which results in most PET investigations giving an effective dose of 5–8 mSv, similar to many CT procedures.

In PET/CT, the dose from the CT component is procedure-dependent. Many centres use a low-dose CT protocol as the images are for attenuation correction and lesion localisation only. Oncology patients will generally be undergoing numerous other CT examinations for disease staging and response assessment, so keeping the dose from the PET examination lower is beneficial. However, most PET/CT systems are capable of full diagnostic-quality CT examinations, so these examinations can be combined if the clinicians feel it would be beneficial to the patient.

Staff and Public

The dose to department staff and the public is purely due to the annihilation radiation (i.e., the 511-keV photons emitted by the patient). Therefore, all areas of the PET facility require significantly increased shielding compared to a standard nuclear medicine department. PET radiopharmacies and imaging rooms are designated as controlled areas and are subject to the requirements for these under the IRR17 legislation. Most PET centres are fitted with ambient dose-rate monitoring systems which will produce an alarm in the event of any significant spillage of radioactivity.

All environmental emissions such as gaseous releases and solid and liquid waste are monitored. The levels of these must be predicted and a licence obtained from the appropriate environmental regulatory body that covers these expected levels. These bodies will also carry out periodic site inspections and investigations of any unexpected releases.

To ensure compliance with the IR(ME)R regulations and to optimise staff safety, all staff should wear personal dosimeters and minimise their time spent close to patients. Pregnant staff should be precluded from working in PET to ensure foetal radiation exposure is minimised. Automated injector systems are now becoming more common in PET as they reduce staff exposure and especially minimise finger doses from the handling of active syringes. These also simplify the use of weight-based dose regimes and can increase patient throughput by more efficiently utilising a fixed production amount of FDG.

REFERENCES

1. Samei E, others. *Assessment of Display Performance for Medical Imaging Systems, Report of the American Association of Physicists in Medicine (AAPM) Task Group 18*. Madison: Medical Physics Publishing; 2005. Available at: https://deckard.duhs.duke.edu/~samei/samei_tg18/index.html (Accessed on: 06 Aug 2022).

2. Administration of Radioactive Substances Advisory Committee. *Notes for Guidance on the Clinical Administration of Radiopharmaceuticals and Use of Sealed Radioactive Sources*; 2021 [Online]. Available at: https://assets.publishing.service.gov.uk/government/uploads/system/uploads/attachment_data/file/961343/ARSAC_NfG_Feb2021.pdf (Accessed on: 06 Aug 2022).

3. UK Statutory Instruments. *The Ionising Radiation (Medical Exposure) Regulations 2017*; 2017 [Online]. Available at: https://www.legislation.gov.uk/uksi/2017/1322/contents/made (Accessed on: 03 Jun 2022).

4. Bolch WE and others: MIRD Pamphlet No. 21: A Generalized Schema for Radiopharmaceutical Dosimetry. *J Nucl Med.* 2009;50:477–484.

5. UK Statutory Instruments. *The Ionising Radiations Regulations 2017*; 2017 [Online]. Available at: https://www.legislation.gov.uk/uksi/2017/1075/contents/made (Accessed on: 03 Jun 2022).

6

Magnetic Resonance Imaging

CHAPTER CONTENTS

MAGNETIC RESONANCE (MR) IMAGING (MRI) SAFETY AND HARDWARE

Guidance and Responsibilities

The main safety guidelines for MR in the UK are *The Safety Guidelines for Magnetic Resonance Imaging Equipment in Clinical Use* produced by the Medicines and Healthcare Regulatory Agency (MHRA).[1] These should be read in conjunction with the department's local rules.

Radiologists play a key role in MRI safety. Only by understanding the risks involved are they able to make an informed choice about the appropriate scan for a patient.

Other key roles in MRI safety are defined by the MHRA guidelines:[1]

MR Responsible Person: Responsible for the day-to-day MR safety (e.g., by ensuring compliance with the MRI local rules).

MR Safety Expert: Provides scientific advice to the MR Responsible Person. Usually a clinical scientist.

Cryogens

MRI scanners either use permanent, resistive, or superconducting magnets. Most clinical MRI scanners use a superconducting magnet design, as permanent and resistive magnets are limited on the magnetic-field strength they can achieve.

In superconducting magnets, a cryogen, usually liquid helium, is used to cool the magnet coils down to near absolute zero. At this temperature, there is no electrical resistance in the coils, which allows a very large current to be passed through them. This creates the strong magnetic field needed for MRI.

Once the magnetic field is created, it is always present, and so the hazards associated with the strong magnetic field are always there. The magnetic field is only switched off in the event of a quench. A quench is a rare occurrence and can either be spontaneous or initiated by the user by pressing the quench button. During a quench, the liquid helium turns into a gas and is vented out of the scanner via the quench pipe. This gas is extremely cold and can displace oxygen, making it potentially dangerous. The MRI scan room is fitted with an oxygen monitor to detect any helium leaks into the room. The quench pipe must be carefully designed to ensure it is able to safely vent the helium out of the building to atmosphere in the event of a quench.

A new design of MRI scanners utilises a very small volume of helium which is permanently sealed inside the magnet, removing the need for a quench pipe, and eliminating the hazards associated with cryogens.

Static Magnetic Field (B_0)

The main magnet (B_0) used in an MRI scanner needs to be very strong. Most clinical MRI scanners are either 1.5 T or 3 T, although some higher-field-strength (e.g., 7 T) and lower-field-strength scanners exist (typically extremity and open scanners). An example MRI scanner is shown in Fig. 6.1.

Scanners can have a wide range of gantry lengths, typically in the range of 125 to 215 cm and are usually 60 or 70 cm wide. Shorter, wider designs offer greater patient comfort and compliance, especially for claustrophobic and larger patients. It is, however, easier to create a large homogeneous field of view (FOV) when using longer, narrower bore designs.

When a patient is exposed to strong magnetic fields, they may experience biological effects such as vertigo, nausea, and a metallic taste. These effects are transient and more pronounced at higher field strengths. Rapid head movement close to the scanner bore should be avoided as this can enhance these sensory effects.

Additional shielding coils are used to ensure that the magnetic field rapidly decreases as you move away from the MRI scanner. This magnetic field is referred to as the fringe field and can interfere with electronic devices.

The MHRA guidelines[1] define two areas, as shown in Fig. 6.2:

MR Environment: The volume surrounding the MRI scanner which contains both the 0.5 mT magnetic-field contour and the Faraday shielded volume. Within this region, items may pose a hazard from exposure to the electromagnetic fields associated with the MRI scanner. Suitable signage should warn of the hazards, and all persons must be appropriately screened before entering.

MR Controlled Access Area: This area is designed to restrict access to the MR Environment. It must contain the MR Environment. Access must be restricted, and suitable warning signs should be displayed at all entrances.

All patients, staff, and volunteers must be verbally screened before entering the MR Controlled Access Area, and fully screened usually using a written screening form before entering the MR Environment. Any implant or metallic foreign body identified by this screening must be reviewed by an authorised member of staff before entering the MR Environment. The MHRA guidelines describe different levels of authorisation for staff working in MRI.[1]

The strong magnetic field can turn loose ferromagnetic objects into projectiles. Several accidents highlight how serious the consequences of this can be.[2,3] Items are classified using the following internationally recognised terminology:[1]

MR Safe: An item which poses no known hazard from exposure to any MR Environment. MR-Safe items are composed of materials that are electrically non-conductive, nonmetallic, and nonmagnetic.

MR Conditional: An item with demonstrated safety in the MR Environment within defined conditions. The conditions must address the static magnetic field, the switched gradient magnetic field, and the radio-frequency (RF) fields. Additional conditions, including specific configurations of the item, may be required.

MR Unsafe: Any item which poses an unacceptable risk to the patient, medical staff, or other persons within the MR Environment.

In addition, the MHRA guidelines describe items as **MR Unlabelled** when there is no safety information available.[1] These items require a risk assessment before entering the MR Environment.

Ferromagnetic objects will also experience a rotational force, called torque, as items try to align themselves along the magnetic-field lines. Some old aneurysm clips are ferromagnetic, and the torque force applied to these has resulted in at least one patient death.[4]

When a conductive material is moved through a magnetic field, the change in magnetic field induces a

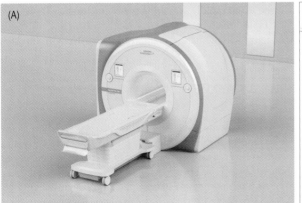
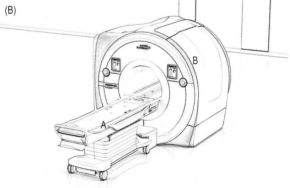

Fig. 6.1 Magnetic resonance imaging (MRI) scanner. *A*, Patient table; *B*, MRI gantry. (Credit Siemens Healthcare Ltd.)

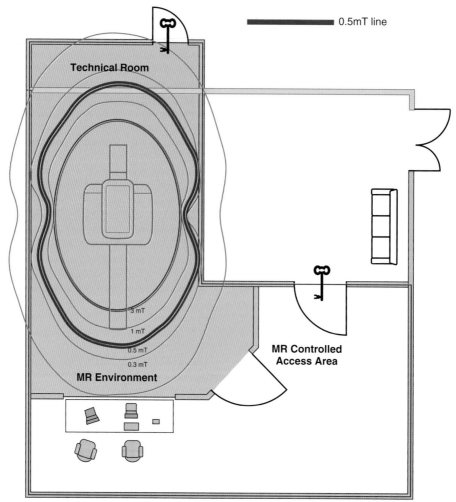

━━━━━━━━━━ 0.5mT line

Technical Room

3 mT
1 mT
0.5 mT
0.3 mT

MR Environment

MR Controlled
Access Area

Fig. 6.2 Diagram showing a typical layout for a magnetic resonance (MR) imaging suite, showing the MR Environment and MR Controlled Access Area.

current in the conductor. The associated magnetic field will oppose the initial changing magnetic field. This is Lenz's law, and the currents produced are referred to as eddy currents. The forces acting on implants due to this effect are considered negligible up to 3 T.

Time-Varying Magnetic Fields (dB/dt)

During scanning, patients are exposed to time-varying magnetic fields. These arise from the gradient coils, which are used to spatially encode the MR signal. The rapid change in magnetic field can induce electrical currents within the patient. These may interfere with the normal function of nerve and muscle cells and can result in peripheral nerve stimulation (PNS). PNS is more likely when using rapidly switching gradients, such as those used in rapid imaging techniques like cardiac and diffusion imaging. Gradients are defined by their strength and slew rate (Fig. 6.3):

$$Slew\ rate = \frac{Peak\ Gradient\ Amplitude}{Rise\ Time}$$

Time-varying magnetic fields also cause heating and vibration of implanted devices due to Lenz's law. Heating caused by gradients is typically much less than the heating caused by RF pulses.

As alternating currents are passed through the gradient coils, forces are exerted on the gradient coils causing them to move. This rapid movement creates acoustic noise,

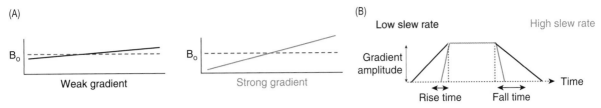

Fig. 6.3 (A) Gradient strength (typically 30–50 mT/m). (B) Slew rate (typically up to 200 T/m/s).

which can reach very high levels. Patients and anyone else remaining in the room during the scan are therefore required to wear hearing protection to ensure they are not exposed to noise levels above 85 dB(A).[1]

RF Pulses (B₁)

The MR signal is produced by applying RF pulses to the body. RF coils are used to transmit and receive these RF signals. One such RF coil is built into the scanner housing and is typically used to transmit the RF signal. This means that the whole volume of the patient that is within the bore of the magnet is exposed to the RF pulses. Local coils placed close to the anatomy of interest are then used to detect the signal and are chosen to be as close to the anatomy of interest as possible to improve the signal-to-noise ratio (SNR). The MRI scanner is placed within a Faraday cage, so that only RF signal originating from the patient is detected.

RF pulses cause heating. A temperature increase of 1°C is typically tolerated by a healthy patient. The actual heat stress experienced by a patient will depend on many factors such as MRI sequence type and parameters, the patient's thermoregulatory response, ambient room temperature, humidity, and air flow. At higher field strength, more energy is required to achieve the same RF pulse, and so RF heating typically increases.

Specific absorption rate (SAR): Used to estimate the rate at which RF energy is being absorbed by tissues during MRI scanning. Different modes are set on the MRI scanner to limit temperature rise, as shown in Table 6.1.

B₁+RMS: This is an alternative method of measuring how much RF will be deposited in a patient. This measure has the advantage that it is independent of patient characteristics and can be calculated in advance of the scan.

Specific energy dose (SED): SED is a measure of the total energy deposited into the patient during an MRI scan. Some scanners may provide warnings or prevent scanning if an SED threshold is reached.

In addition to heat stress of the patient, localised heating can occur resulting in burns. There have been several cases reported where inappropriate peripheral

TABLE 6.1 Modes of Operation for SAR Recommended in the Medicines and Healthcare Products Regulatory Agency[1] Guidelines

Mode	Maximum Whole-Body Temperature Rise (°C)	Whole-Body SAR Limit (W/kg)
Normal mode	0.5	2
First level (controlled)	1.0	4
Research	>1.0	>4

SAR, specific absorption rate.

equipment has been connected to a patient, resulting in significant localised heating leading to patient burns.[2,5] Heating is also a concern for patients with implants, as the tissue surrounding the implant can heat up. MR Conditional implants may give a SAR limit which needs to be met to ensure heating is within acceptable limits.

Transmit/Receive (Tx/Rx) Coils

Some local coils both transmit and receive the MR signal. The advantage of local-coil RF transmission is that only the anatomy enclosed within the transmit coil experiences the RF pulse. Any anatomy outside of the coil does not experience heating and does not contribute to the image. The knee coil is usually a Tx/Rx coil to prevent the other knee being excited and aliasing into the image. Some implants are MR Conditional, with a condition that only imaging with a specific Tx/Rx coil is permitted.

Phased-Array Coils

The signal from a single coil element is high close to the coil, but rapidly drops off as the distance away from the coil increases (Fig. 6.4). Larger coils can increase coverage, but most modern coils use phased-array coils to create a uniform

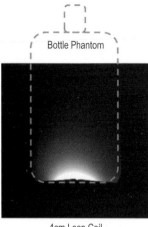

Bottle Phantom

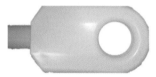

4cm Loop Coil

Fig. 6.4 Signal from a single coil element. Signal is high close to the coil, but rapidly drops off with distance.

image with high signal across a large FOV. Phased-array coils use multiple independent elements with known sensitivities that can be combined to create a single image (Fig. 6.5).

Regular quality assurance (QA) should be used to check whether any elements are not functioning within a phased-array coil.

Phased-array coils are essential for parallel imaging techniques.

Implants

The safety status of all implants should be determined before a patient enters the MR Environment. Implants can be active (e.g. pacemaker) or passive (e.g. stent). Although most modern implants are MR Safe or MR Conditional, it is essential that all implants are known about and reviewed before a patient is scanned.

The MHRA guidelines[1] provide advice for how to proceed if a patient needs to be scanned outside of the conditions given by the manufacturer (off-label). For instance, if the safety status is unknown (e.g. a metallic foreign body is present), the patient has an MR-Unsafe device fitted or the MR conditions cannot be met. In these situations, the MRI scan may still be able to take

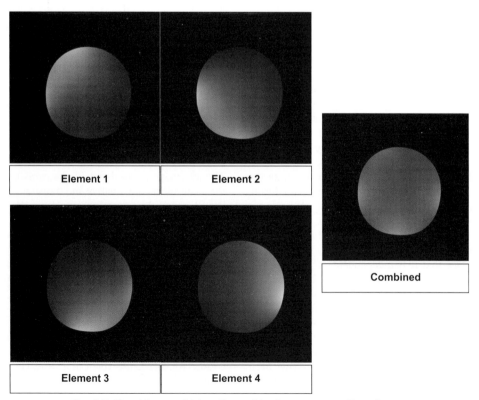

Element 1   Element 2

Combined

Element 3   Element 4

Fig. 6.5 Signal from multiple coils combined to create a uniform image.

place if a risk assessment demonstrates that the benefit to the patient outweighs the risks, and steps to mitigate the risks are taken.

Contrast Agents

Gadolinium-based contrast agents (GBCAs) are regularly administered in MRI to provide additional information, but they do carry risks. It has been shown that there is a link between nephrogenic systemic fibrosis (NSF) and gadolinium administration for patients with poor renal function. Steps should be taken to minimise risks, such as identification of patients with poor renal function who may not be suitable for contrast[6]. Not all GBCAs carry the same level of risk of NSF. GBCAs are categorised as macrocyclic or linear depending on their chemical structure. Macrocyclic contrast agents are thought to carry a lower risk than linear ones as they are more stable. The lowest risk agent which gives the clinical information should be used.

More recently, gadolinium deposition in tissues including the brain has been observed.[7] At the time of writing, there is no strong evidence to confirm that there are harmful effects associated with the accumulation of gadolinium in the body. However, several linear contrast agents have been suspended from use in Europe as a precautionary measure.[8]

Pregnant Patients

The pregnancy status for all patients should be established during screening. There is no clear evidence that MRI is harmful to the foetus.[1] Evidence surrounding RF and noise exposure is limited and therefore it is prudent to minimise exposure to these. If a patient is pregnant, then a radiologist should take this into consideration when deciding whether the scan is justified. If justified, the scan should proceed at the lowest available field strength and all reasonable steps should be taken to reduce exposure to acoustic noise and RF. Scans should be undertaken in normal operating mode wherever possible, and the use of GBCAs should be avoided unless a radiologist agrees that the administration is absolutely necessary.[6]

SIGNAL CREATION, DETECTION, AND LOCALISATION

Signal Origin

Any nuclei with an odd number of protons will exhibit nuclear MR. However, most clinical MRI uses hydrogen because it has a large magnetic moment and is abundant in

the body in many different chemical environments. Other nuclei, such as ^{13}C, ^{129}Xe, ^{3}He, and ^{31}P, are the subject of research but at the time of writing are not widely used clinically.

Each hydrogen atom has a single positively charged proton. Each proton spins on its own axis, and therefore in MRI these are commonly referred to as spins. Each spin acts like a tiny magnet and so has a magnetic moment associated with it.

In the absence of an external magnetic field, all the spins are aligned randomly. Their magnetic moments cancel out so there is no net magnetisation. If an external magnetic field (B_0) is applied, then these spins will align either parallel or antiparallel to the applied magnetic field (Fig. 6.6). Slightly more spins will align with B_0 rather than against it, and so a net magnetisation (M_0) will be produced.

M_0 increases with increasing field strength, so higher-field-strength scanners typically have a higher SNR. By convention, the axis along the length of the MRI scanner is referred to as the z-axis, and so this magnetisation is said to be in the z direction ($M_z = M_0$).

The spins cannot align exactly to B_0, but rather they precess about the z-axis (Fig. 6.7).

The frequency (ω_0) at which the spins precess is proportional to the applied magnetic field and the gyromagnetic ratio of the element (γ) (for hydrogen, this is 42.6 MHz/T). This frequency is known as the Larmor frequency and is described by this key equation:

$$\omega_0 = \gamma B_0$$

Although the spins are precessing at the same frequency, they will be out of phase with one another as shown in Fig. 6.8.

The net magnetisation at 1.5 T is around 75,000 times smaller than B_0 (which is also in the z-axis).[9] The net magnetisation is therefore swamped by B_0 and cannot be

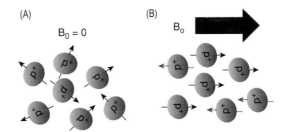

Fig. 6.6 (A) In the absence of a magnetic field, spins do not show a preferred direction. (B) When an external magnetic field (B_0) is applied, spins align with or against B_0, with a net magnetic moment parallel to B_0.

(A)   (B)

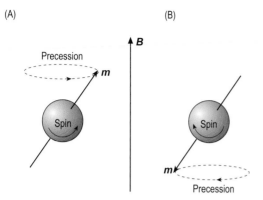

Fig. 6.7 Spins precess about B_0 in one of two states, (A) parallel (spin-up) or (B) antiparallel (spin down).

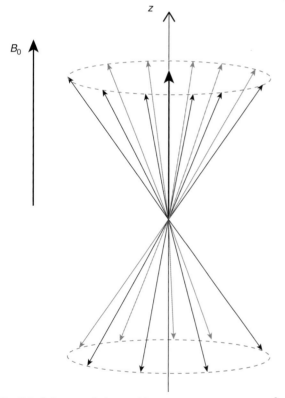

Fig. 6.8 Spins out of phase with one another at equilibrium[9].

detected if left in the z direction. To be able to detect this, it needs to be in the x-y plane.

Resonance

A RF pulse is applied to the spins using an RF transmit coil. The frequency of the RF pulse is set so that it resonates with the spins (i.e., the Larmor frequency).

In a simple spin-echo (SE) pulse sequence, the RF excitation pulse is a 90° RF pulse. The RF pulse rotates the magnetisation from the z plane into the x-y plane. It also causes all the spins to precess in phase with each other. The result is that immediately after the 90° RF pulse, $M_z = 0$ and $M_{xy} = M_0$ (Fig. 6.9).

The magnetisation in the x-y plane, M_{xy}, or free induction decay (FID) can be detected by an RF receive coil. The precessing magnetic field generates a voltage in the RF coils. This is a measurable signal and is at the Larmor frequency.

Flip Angle

By varying the RF pulse strength and duration, other flip angles can be achieved (Fig. 6.10). A 180° pulse will completely invert the magnetisation and is called an inversion pulse (Fig. 6.11).

Signal Localisation

The next step is to localise the signal. Fig. 6.12 shows a basic pulse sequence diagram. In each step, magnetic-field gradients are used to localise the signal.

Slice Selection

The first stage is slice selection. A gradient is applied in the slice direction, causing the magnetic field to vary along this axis. This gradient is applied during the initial RF excitation pulse. Spins that experience a slightly higher magnetic field will precess faster, whereas spins that experience a slightly lower magnetic field will precess slower. The RF excitation pulse can be tuned to only excite spins within a specific frequency range, and therefore only excite spins within a given slice. The thickness of the slice excited will depend on the gradient (G_{SS}) applied, the gyromagnetic ratio, and the transmitter bandwidth (range of frequencies) of the RF pulse:

$$Slice\ Thickness = \frac{Transmitter\ Bandwidth}{\gamma G_{SS}}$$

Artefact: Cross-Talk

The actual slice-selection pulse shape is not perfect. Cross-talk arises when spins in overlapping slices are excited twice (Fig. 6.13). This causes signal reduction. The solution to this is to use a gap between slices or interleave the acquisition so that adjacent slices are not acquired close together. The use of large slice gaps should be avoided, as

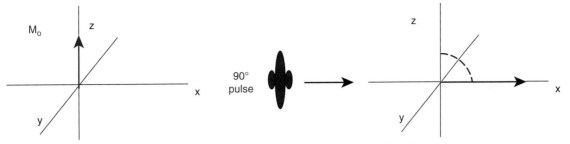

Fig. 6.9 M_O is tipped from the z-axis into the x-y plane using a 90° radiofrequency pulse.

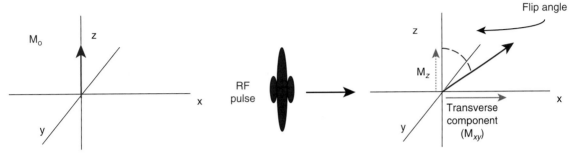

Fig. 6.10 The flip angle will depend on the duration and strength of the applied radiofrequency pulse.

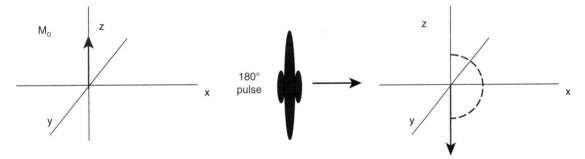

Fig. 6.11 A 180° inversion pulse.

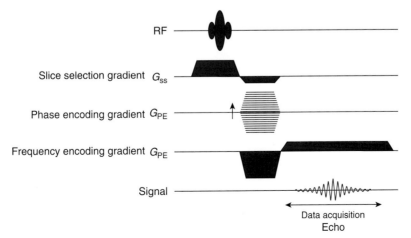

Fig. 6.12 Basic pulse sequence diagram showing the gradients used for spatial encoding. The negative gradients are used to correct for the dephasing caused by the encoding gradients[9].

(A)

One slice

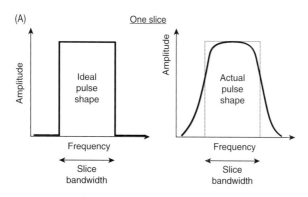

(B)

Multiple slices - cross-talk

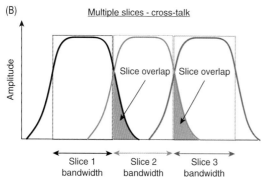

(C)

Multiple slices – slice gap

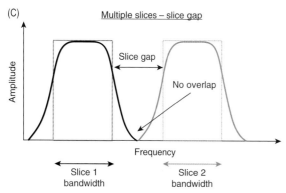

Fig. 6.13 (A) Ideal radiofrequency (RF) pulse shape vs actual RF pulse shape. (B) Slice overlap. (C) Using a slice gap can reduce cross-talk artefacts.

this results in tissue not being imaged, which could result in small pathologies being missed.

Frequency Encoding

To encode the signal in the second direction, a further gradient is applied perpendicular to the first, this time during signal readout. This gradient causes the frequency of the detected signal to vary with position. These different

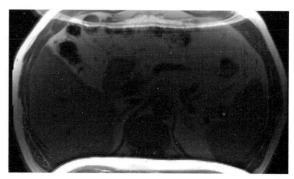

Fig. 6.14 Aliasing artefact. Phase encoding is anteroposterior.

frequencies can then be separated out using a mathematic technique called a Fourier transform. The receiver bandwidth is the range of frequencies received during signal readout.

Phase Encoding

To get information from the third axis, a third gradient is applied perpendicular to the other two gradients in between excitation and readout. Switching this gradient on and off again induces a spatially dependent phase shift. It is not possible to separate out the different phases using a single measurement, so this phase encoding is repeated many times to localise the signal in this direction.

Artefact: Wrap/Aliasing

Aliasing is a common image artefact that can be avoided by careful planning of images. During phase encoding, it is impossible for tissues with a phase shift of 361° to be distinguished from those with a phase shift of 1°. Therefore, tissues outside of the FOV can appear wrapped into the image (Fig. 6.14).

Multislice Imaging

To acquire multiple slices, the dead time between signal acquisition and the next RF excitation pulse is used to acquire signal from different slices.

2D vs 3D

2D scans typically have good in-plane resolution, but poor slice resolution. This means they cannot be reconstructed into other planes. 2D images can suffer from partial volume effects. Small pathologies may be missed if the slice thickness is too large for the anatomy being imaged.

In 3D imaging, the whole imaging volume is excited with the initial RF excitation pulse. Additional phase-encoding gradients are then applied to obtain the additional positional information. This results in long acquisition times. Voxels can be isotropic, so resolution is good in all planes, allowing the data to be reconstructed into any plane.

BASIC IMAGE CONTRAST MECHANISMS

Relaxation

Immediately after the initial RF excitation pulse, two independent effects occur: spin-lattice (T_1) relaxation and spin-spin (T_2) relaxation.

T_1 Relaxation

The RF excitation pulse moves the spins into an excited state. After this excitation, the spins exchange energy with the surrounding tissue (lattice) to move back to their equilibrium state. This is the recovery of M_0 in the z-axis and is exponential (Fig. 6.15). Spins which exchange energy efficiently with their surrounding tissue have a short T_1 relaxation time. The T_1 time of a tissue is when 63% of the initial magnetisation has recovered.

In T_1-weighted (T_1w) images, tissues with short T_1 (e.g., fat) recover signal very quickly and have high signal. Tissues with longer T_1 values (e.g., cerebrospinal fluid [CSF]) recover slowly and have lower signal.

It is easy to get good contrast between tissues with different T_1 relaxation times, so T_1w images are used for high-resolution anatomical imaging.

T_2 Relaxation

Immediately after the RF excitation pulse, spins are in phase with each other, and so for a 90° RF excitation pulse, $M_{xy} = M_0$. Random spin-spin interactions mean that each spin experiences a slightly different local magnetic field, and therefore precess at a slightly different rate. The spins become out of phase, and M_{xy} reduces exponentially (Fig. 6.16) as the spins cancel each other out. Spins which tumble more slowly interact more with neighbouring spins, and therefore have a shorter T_2 relaxation time. The T_2 relaxation time of a tissue is the time for M_{xy} to drop to 37% of the initial magnetisation.

In T_2-weighted (T_2w) images tissues with short T_2 (e.g., solids) dephase quickly and therefore appear as low signal. Tissues with longer T_2 values (e.g., fluid) dephase slower and appear as bright signal.

T_2w images are useful to demonstrate pathology, as this is often associated with fluid accumulation.

T_2* Relaxation

In addition to random spin-spin interactions, dephasing of the spins and therefore reduction of M_{xy} occurs due to inhomogeneities in the magnetic field and magnetic susceptibility at the interfaces between tissues. T_2* describes relaxation due to all these effects.

Proton Density (PD)

Different tissues have slightly different proton densities, and therefore different M_0. Tissues with higher water content have a higher PD and appear bright on PD-weighted (PDw) images. The range of PDs is quite narrow, so PDw images lack contrast. PDw images are frequently used in musculoskeletal imaging.

Contrast

Contrast-enhanced imaging is achieved through the administration of GBCAs. Gadolinium is paramagnetic,

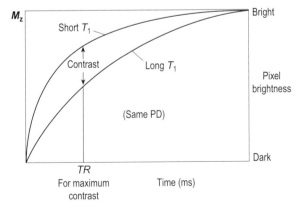

Fig. 6.15 T_1 relaxation. To maximise T_1 contrast, use a short TR (repetition time).

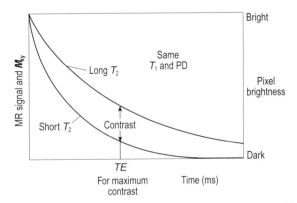

Fig. 6.16 T_2 relaxation. To maximise T_2 contrast use a long TE (echo time).

which means it becomes temporarily magnetised when placed in an external magnetic field and aligns with the external magnetic field. Tissues where gadolinium accumulates have a reduced T_1 relaxation time, and therefore appear brighter on T_1w images. Gadolinium also causes a mild reduction in T_2, but this is generally only noticeable on clinical images where the concentration of gadolinium is high.

Other Contrast Agents

It is possible to use other natural contrast agents to change the appearance of MRI images. For instance, pineapple juice can be used to reduce the signal from the gastrointestinal tract when performing MR cholangiopancreatography. Pineapple juice contains manganese which acts to reduce T_2 and causes signal to decrease on T_2w images.

BASIC MRI SEQUENCES

MRI pulse sequences can broadly be split into two main groups: spin echo (SE) and gradient echo (GRE).

Spin Echo (SE) Sequence

A simple SE sequence utilises two RF pulses, an initial 90° RF excitation pulse, and a 180° refocusing pulse (Fig. 6.17). The 180° pulse creates the echo, and rephases some of the T_2^* dephasing, so that only the random T_2 relaxation affects the contrast in the final image.

Echo time (TE) is the time between the initial 90° RF pulse and the signal readout. The 180° refocusing pulse occurs at TE/2.

Repetition time (TR) is the time between two subsequent excitation pulses.

In a simple SE sequence, different image weightings can be achieved by varying TE and TR. Figs. 6.15 and 6.16 show how TE and TR can be utilised to maximise image contrast in T_1w and T_2w images. Table 6.2 gives example parameters to achieve different image contrast.

The scan time for a basic SE sequence can be calculated from:

TABLE 6.2 Example Parameters for Spin-Echo Sequences

	TE	TR
T_1w	Short (<30 ms)	Short (300–800 ms)
T_2w	Long (>80 ms)	Long (>2000 ms)
PDw	Short (<30 ms)	Long (>1000 ms)

PDw, proton density-weighted imaging; TE, echo time; TR, repetition time; T_1w, T_1-weighted imaging; T_2w, T_2-weighted imaging.

$$Scan\ time = TR \times N_{PE} \times NSA$$

where N_{PE} is the number of phase-encoding steps, and NSA (or NEX) is the number of averages.

Fast or Turbo SE (FSE or TSE)

To speed up sequences, more than one echo can be acquired per TR. Multiple 180° refocussing pulses with different phase-encoding gradients are applied within each TR. For instance, if an echo train length (ETL) or turbo factor (TF) of 3 is used, acquisition time would reduce by one-third. The use of multiple large RF pulses in a short space of time causes these sequences to have high SAR. Motion artefacts are likely to be reduced as the imaging time is reduced.

In TSE, signals are acquired with different TEs. The overall contrast of the image will be determined by the effective TE, which is the TE used to fill the centre of k-space.

Using sequences with a long ETL results in increased T_2 weighting, as the effective TE will increase. The later echoes will have a lower signal, which can lead to a loss of spatial resolution if these are used to fill the outer parts of k-space.

Single-Shot TSE (SS-TSE)

SS-TSE sequences are very quick sequences often used in breath-hold studies. This sequence uses a single excitation

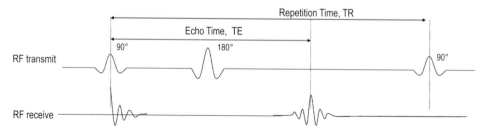
Fig. 6.17 Simple spin-echo sequence.

pulse followed by a long echo train so that all data for a given slice is acquired within one TR. The effective TE is long, due to the long ETL. The Half Fourier Single-Shot Turbo spin echo (HASTE) sequence combines half Fourier with SS-TSE to produce heavily T_2w images frequently used in abdominal imaging.

Multiecho

By applying two refocusing pulses after the initial excitation pulse, it is possible to generate two images with different echo times. Images with two different weightings can be produced (e.g., a PDw and T_2w image).

Gradient Echo (GRE) Sequences

GRE sequences are typically much faster than SE sequences and are essential in areas where rapid imaging is required (e.g., cardiovascular imaging).[10] They usually have a lower SNR compared to SE sequences and are more likely to suffer with artefacts.

In GRE, there is no $180°$ refocussing pulse. Instead, gradients are used to dephase and then rephase the signal to create an echo. Images are no longer T_2w, but instead will be T_2^*w, as the effects of magnetic-field inhomogeneities and magnetic susceptibilities are not rephased.

The RF excitation pulse is typically smaller than $90°$. Not all M_z is tipped into the x-y plane. The residual magnetisation in the z-axis means that the TR can be reduced, as the time required for T_1 recovery is shortened.

The flip angle and TE control the image contrast. Example parameters are given in Table 6.3.

Spoiled-Gradient Echo

Spoiling aims to remove any remaining signal in the x-y plane after each cycle so that it does not contribute to the next image acquisition. Either a gradient is applied at the end of the cycle to dephase any signal remaining in the x-y plane (gradient spoiling) or a phase shift is applied to the RF excitation pulse (RF spoiling).

TABLE 6.3 Example Parameters for Gradient-Echo Sequences

	TE	Flip Angle
T_1w	Short (<30 ms)	Large >70°
T_2^*w	Long (>80 ms)	Small 5–20°
PDw	Short (<30 ms)	Small 5–20°

PDw, proton density-weighted imaging; *TE*, echo time; *T_1w*, T_1-weighted imaging; *T_2^*w*, T_2^*-weighted imaging.

Steady-State Free Precision

If the TR is short and no spoiling is utilised, then the residual transverse magnetisation can carry over to the next TR and contribute to the signal. To maximise the signal, the gradients are rewound to bring the signal back into phase. This increases the signal but results in a more complex tissue contrast that relates to the ratio of T_1/T_2.

BEYOND THE BASIC SEQUENCES

Echo Planar Imaging (EPI)

EPI is an extremely fast imaging sequence useful for techniques that require many rapidly acquired images, like diffusion and functional MRI (fMRI). All data is acquired within a single TR. An initial echo is created (either using a SE or GRE technique) and followed by a series of gradient echoes to fill k-space within a single TR. This sequence is low-resolution, has a low SNR, and suffers from chemical-shift and susceptibility artefacts.

Fat Saturation (FS)

Due to their different chemical environments, the resonant frequency of fat and water are not the same. There is a chemical shift of 3.5 parts per million (ppm) between fat and water.

In FS, unwanted fat signal is removed by applying an RF pulse immediately before the sequence with a narrow transmitter bandwidth that is only resonant with fat protons. Only the fat protons are excited by this RF pulse. A gradient is then applied to dephase or spoil the fat signal so that it does not contribute to the image. FS relies on good magnetic-field homogeneity so that the fat peak can be separated from the water peak (Fig. 6.18). FS tends to fail for large FOVs and near metal implants.

FS is easier to achieve at higher field strength because there is a greater separation between the fat and water peak (220 Hz at 1.5 T, compared to 440 Hz at 3 T).

Artefact: Chemical Shift (Spatial Misregistration)

The chemical shift between fat and water causes problems for frequency encoding. Fat signal can appear shifted in the frequency-encoding direction (Fig. 6.19). This artefact is more severe at higher field strength and when the receiver bandwidth is low.

Artefact: Chemical Shift (Phase Cancellation)

In GRE, any voxel which contains both fat and water will have a signal which varies with TE. These voxels are

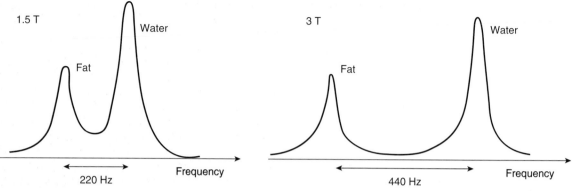

Fig. 6.18 The difference in resonance frequency between fat and water is the chemical shift.

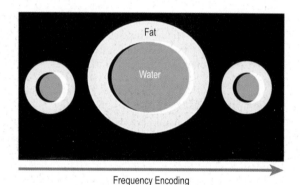

Fig. 6.19 Chemical-shift misregistration artefact.

typically at the interfaces between tissues. Images acquired when the fat and water are completely out of phase with each other will have low signal in these voxels. This can appear as a dark outline around organs (Fig. 6.20B). Phase cancellation can be overcome by acquiring at a different TE, e.g., when the fat and water spins are in phase.

Dixon Imaging

Dixon imaging uses GRE images with different TEs. In-phase (IP) and out-of-phase (OP) images are acquired and then processed to produce fat-suppressed and water-suppressed images (Fig. 6.20).

The signal in each voxel is:

$$S_{IP} = S_{water} + S_{fat}$$

$$S_{OP} = S_{water} - S_{fat}$$

$S_{water} = 0.5(S_{OP} + S_{IP})$; i.e., water signals add, fat signals cancel out

$S_{fat} = 0.5(S_{OP} - S_{IP})$; i.e., fat signals add, water signals cancel out

Artefact: Dixon Artefact

Fig. 6.21 shows an artefact caused by a computation error where the fat and water are swapped, so fat-suppressed images show bright fat and water-suppressed images show bright fluid. This can affect the whole image, or just a region within an image.

Inversion Recovery (IR)

IR techniques are used to remove the signal from a given tissue type. A 180° inversion pulse is applied before a standard image sequence. This tips M_z into the negative z direction. An inversion time (TI) is then allowed for T_1 recovery to occur. When the given tissue has recovered to zero magnetisation in the z plane, the excitation pulse is applied. This tissue has no magnetisation to be tipped and therefore does not contribute to the final image. The exact TI time will depend on the T_1 of the tissue and the chosen TR (Fig. 6.22).

FLAIR: Fluid attenuation IR, uses a long TI to null signal from fluid.

STIR: Short TI IR, uses a short TI to null signal from fat.

SPIR: Spectral IR, uses a 180° inversion pulse that is tuned to excite only fat protons. SNR is improved compared to STIR, but this technique relies on good magnetic-field homogeneity so that only the fat protons are inverted.

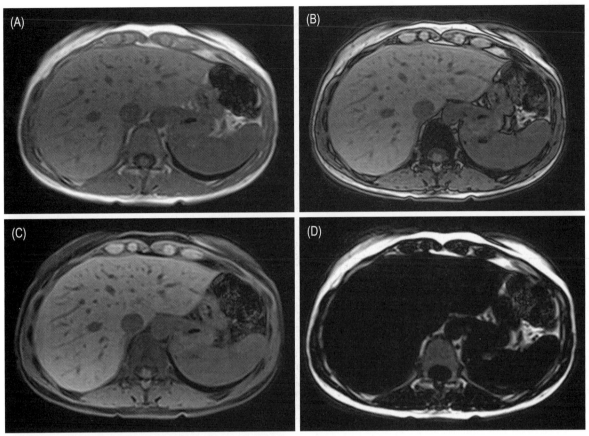

Fig. 6.20 Dixon imaging. (A) In phase, (B) out of phase, (C) water image, (D) fat image.

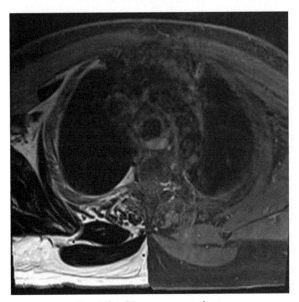

Fig. 6.21 Dixon swap artefact.

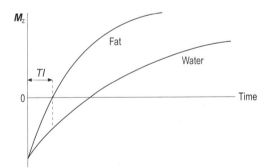

Fig. 6.22 Inversion recovery sequence.

The IR pulse can be added to other sequences to prepare them. One example is the use of a 3D spoiled GRE with an IR pulse (MP-RAGE), which is commonly used in neuroimaging to acquire T_1w images of the brain. The use of the inversion pulse causes the image to be more T_1 weighted.

In double IR (DIR), signal from two different tissues is suppressed by applying two inversion pulses with different TIs. This can be used in neuroimaging to suppress CSF and white matter to allow visualisation of multiple sclerosis plaques.

In cardiac black-blood imaging, two inversion pulses are applied. The first is a non-selective pulse that inverts all the spins. The second is applied rapidly after the first and is slice-selective. Stationary spins such as the myocardium have their spins restored, whereas blood flowing into the slice has been inverted. Careful selection of the TI then allows images with black blood to be acquired.[10,11]

K-SPACE

K-space is where the acquired data is stored and is related to the image via a Fourier transform. Each point in k-space contains frequency and phase information for the entire image. The intensity of each point in k-space reflects how much that spatial frequency contributes to the final image.

The centre of k-space contains the image contrast information, whereas the edge of k-space contains the resolution information (Fig. 6.23).

In the simplest sequence, each phase-encoding step fills one line of k-space (Fig. 6.24). There are many alternative ways to fill k-space, including radial and partial filling (Fig. 6.25). K-space is symmetrical, so it is possible to speed up scans by only acquiring some of the data.

Half or partial Fourier: Some phase-encoding steps are skipped. Missing lines of k-space are synthesised from existing data. For half Fourier, the scan time is nearly 50%, SNR decreases by 30%, and resolution remains unchanged.

Zero filling: The larger phase-encoding steps are not acquired. Missing lines of k-space are filled with zeros. SNR remains unchanged as no signal or noise is added. The resolution can appear increased.

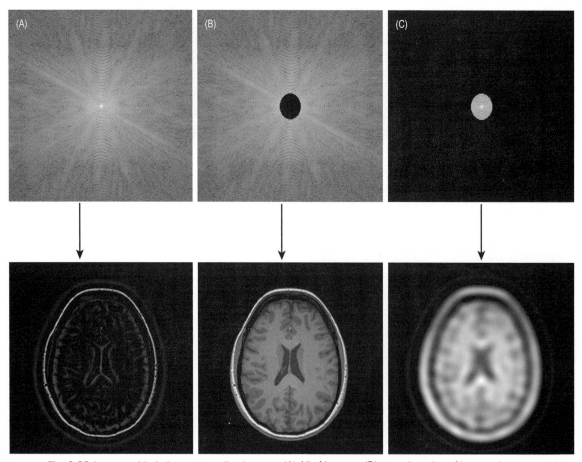

Fig. 6.23 Images with their corresponding k-space. (A) All of k-space, (B) central section of k-space (contrast data) removed, (C) outer edges of k-space (resolution data) removed.

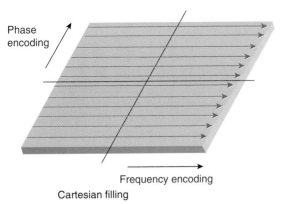

Phase encoding

Frequency encoding

Cartesian filling

Fig. 6.24 Cartesian filling of k-space (line by line).

Partial echo: The first part of the echo is not sampled. The missing data is synthesised from the acquired data. TE and TR can be reduced, allowing acquisition time to be reduced. The SNR is reduced but the resolution remains unchanged.

Radial filling (BLADE/PROPELLER): Reduces motion artefacts by filling k-space radially. The central area of k-space is oversampled and used to correct for in-plane motion.

Compressed sensing (CS): K-space is incompletely filled. The missing datapoints are semi-random to reduce artefacts and are preferentially towards the periphery of k-space to ensure the important contrast information in the centre is kept. The missing datapoints are estimated by iterative reconstruction. This technique works well on sparse data (e.g., MR angiograms), but can be applied to other images if a sparsifying transformation is used.

Artefacts: K-space

A single spike in k-space will appear as bright and dark alternating stripes across the image. This is known as a herringbone or corduroy artefact. This can indicate a problem with the coil or scanner.

IMAGE QUALITY AND SCAN TIME

SNR, Resolution and Scan Time

When acquiring MRI scans, there is usually a compromise between the SNR, resolution, and scan time.

High in-plane spatial resolution is required for most anatomical imaging. Increasing spatial resolution can be achieved either by decreasing the FOV or increasing the matrix size (Fig. 6.26).

Low SNR causes images to appear grainy. SNR can be increased by increasing the voxel volume, increasing the number of signals averaged, or reducing the receiver bandwidth.

A QA programme should be in place to identify any deterioration in image quality which could indicate a problem with the MRI scanner. IPEM Report 112 gives recommendations on QA tests to perform and their frequencies.[12]

Some methods to reduce scan time have already been mentioned; others are discussed here.

Parallel Imaging (SENSE, GRAPPA, iPAT)

Parallel imaging is used to reduce scan times. Parallel imaging utilises the known coil sensitivities of the different elements within a phased-array coil to reduce the number

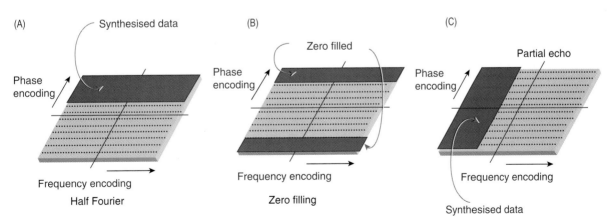

(A) Synthesised data

Phase encoding

Frequency encoding

Half Fourier

(B) Zero filled

Phase encoding

Frequency encoding

Zero filling

(C) Partial echo

Phase encoding

Frequency encoding

Synthesised data

Fig. 6.25 Alternative methods to fill k-space and reduce acquisition time. (A) Half Fourier, (B) zero filling, and (C) partial echo.

(A)   Field of view   (B)   Matrix size

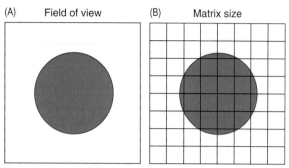

Fig. 6.26 The spatial resolution depends on (A) the field of view and (B) the matrix size.

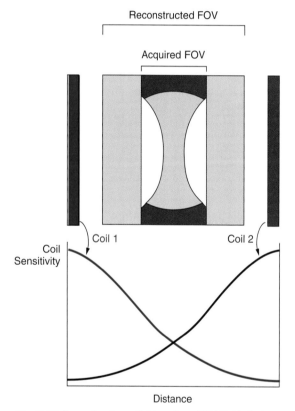

Fig. 6.27 Example of parallel imaging. *FOV,* field of view.

of phase-encoding steps acquired and therefore the acquisition time. Reducing the number of phase-encoding steps results in a reduced FOV and therefore aliasing. The coil sensitivities are then used to unfold the data to get a true representation of the data (Fig. 6.27). If the scan time is reduced by 50%, SNR is reduced to around 70%. The SNR reduction will depend on the geometry or g-factor of

the coil, which is a measure of how well the coil configuration can unwrap the aliasing.

Artefacts: Parallel Imaging

If the acceleration factor is too high, images can appear noisy. In parallel imaging, noise is not evenly distributed across the image, causing some areas to appear noisier than others, depending on the g-factor.

If the reconstructed FOV is too small compared to the imaged object, then aliasing artefacts can arise. In parallel imaging, this appears as ghost signal in the centre of the FOV.

Simultaneous Multislice Imaging (SMS)

SMS can speed up acquisition times, with little reduction in SNR or resolution. In SMS, multiband RF excitation pulses are utilised, which contain multiple different frequencies to excite multiple slices, applying a phase shift between them. Aliased slices are then separated out during image reconstruction.

ARTEFACTS

Some artefacts have already been discussed in their relevant sections. Others are described here. This is not an exhaustive list, as the range of artefacts in MRI is extensive. Other artefacts are described within the references.[9,12,13,14]

Movement

Patient movement causes ghosting and blurring of images. The phase-encoding direction is most affected. Padding can be used to immobilise the patient. The scan time can be reduced for patients who are unable to keep still, but this will usually result in sacrificing either SNR or resolution. Radial k-space techniques can help to reduce movement artefact.

Thoracic and abdominal imaging suffer from physiological motion. Artefacts from breathing can be overcome by scanning with the patient holding their breath, or by acquiring respiratory-gated images where images are acquired at the same point in the breathing cycle. Similarly, cardiac motion can be overcome using cardiac gating. Artefacts from peristalsis can be overcome using antispasmodic drugs.

Truncation (Gibb's)

Truncation artefacts appear at boundaries between bright and dark signal. Alternating lines of bright and dark signal are seen which reduce in intensity away from the boundary. This artefact arises when the matrix size is reduced to speed up a scan and is most commonly seen in the phase-encoding direction. Reducing the matrix size reduces the number of frequencies which are used to create the image, and therefore high-contrast boundaries are not sufficiently represented. The artefact can be reduced by repeating the scan with a higher phase-encoding matrix.

Flow

Moving blood or CSF results in signal void or ghosting artefacts (Fig. 6.28).

In SE sequences, flowing blood may not experience both the 90° and 180° pulses needed to create an echo, so vessels appear dark.

In GRE, only one RF pulse is used. Blood flowing into the slide will have a higher M_z than static tissue. Vessels therefore appear bright and may cause ghosts in the phase-encoding direction. To overcome ghosting, spatial saturation bands can be placed above or below the slice to null signal flowing into the image.

Susceptibility/Metal

Any paramagnetic (e.g., oxygen, iron ions) or ferromagnetic materials (e.g., iron, cobalt, nickel) will cause local magnetic-field distortions, resulting in incorrect frequency encoding and local dephasing. This results in image distortions mainly in the frequency-encoding direction, and areas of signal void. Metal implants will cause the most significant artefacts; however, more subtle susceptibility artefacts will also be seen at interfaces between tissues of different susceptibilities (e.g., skull base).

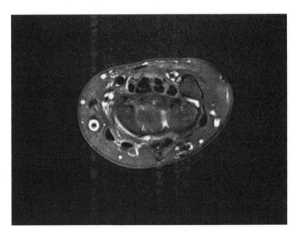

Fig. 6.28 Flow artefact.

These artefacts are less prominent on SE sequences as the 180° refocusing pulse helps to rephase the dephasing caused by magnetic-field inhomogeneities. Where metal implants are within the FOV, GRE- and EPI-based sequences should be avoided where possible.

Reducing TE, increasing receiver bandwidth, and using a lower field strength can all be used to reduce susceptibility artefacts (Fig. 6.29). If fat nulling is required, then STIR will be more reliable than FS.

Modern MRI scanners have dedicated metal artefacts reduction sequences (MARS). It is not possible to completely eliminate metal artefacts, but their effect can be significantly reduced.

Zipper

A line of alternating dark and light signal is called a zipper artefact and is caused by RF interference (Fig. 6.30).

It can be difficult to identify the source of RF. RF interference may arise from problems with the scanner or coils, equipment within the scan room, or a failure of the Faraday cage.

Gradient Nonlinearities

Applied magnetic-field gradients are only linear over a limited range. Gradient non-linearities can result in incorrect spatial encoding at the edges of a large FOV. Scanners have distortion correction software that can be used to compensate for this.

B₁ Inhomogeneities

Dielectric artefacts arise when the wavelength of the RF pulse is similar to the structure being imaged. This can be problematic at 3 T when imaging abdomens, particularly when there is lots of fluid present, and so it is advisable to scan pregnant patients and patients with ascites at 1.5 T.

ADVANCED TECHNIQUES

MR Angiography (MRA)

MRA is split into contrast-enhanced MRA and non-contrast MRA and are often displayed as maximum intensity profile (MIP) images.

Contrast-Enhanced MRA

In contrast-enhanced MRA, a bolus of gadolinium is injected. Images are acquired during the first pass of the

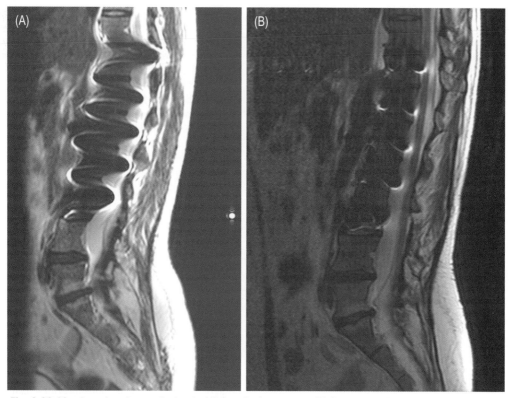

Fig. 6.29 Metal artefact from spinal rods. (A) Standard sequence. (B) Sequence adapted to reduce artefact.

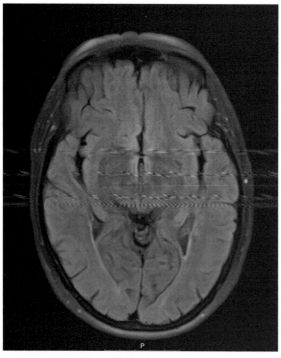

Fig. 6.30 Zipper artefact.

bolus through the vessels of interest. The centre of k-space is acquired as the peak of the bolus passes through the vessels of interest; the outer parts of k-space can be filled after the peak of the contrast. A fast 3D GRE sequence is used, which saturates the signal from static tissue. Contrast agents reduce the T_1 of the surrounding blood, causing it to recover quickly and appear bright.

Time-Resolved MRA

3D MRA images are acquired dynamically before, during, and after the injection of contrast agent. This eliminates any timing issues associated with standard contrast-enhanced MRA, where it is possible to miss the peak of the bolus passing through the vessels of interest. Good temporal resolution is required. To achieve this, the full k-space data is acquired for the first or last acquisition, but only the centre of k-space (containing the contrast information) is acquired during the dynamic acquisition. The periphery of k-space is then filled with the data from the full k-space acquisition. More complex versions of this (e.g., TWIST/TRICKS) also partially acquire peripheral

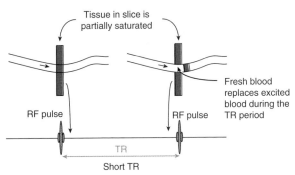

Fig. 6.31 Time-of-flight magnetic resonance angiography. *RF,* radiofrequency; *TR,* repetition time.

data in the dynamic phase, and data is then shared between different timepoints.

Time-of-Flight (TOF) MRA

TOF MRA is a non-contrast technique. A GRE sequence with short TE and TR but a large flip angle is used. Spins which are stationary become saturated and do not contribute significantly to the image. Blood flowing into the slice has not experienced previous RF pulses and so contributes a larger signal to the image, appearing bright (Fig. 6.31). To maximise this effect, slices are acquired perpendicular to the main direction of flow.

Phase-Contrast (PC) MRA

Phase-contrast MRA is another non-contrast technique. A bipolar gradient is applied. Spins which are stationary show no phase change due to the equal and opposite gradients. Spins which are moving experience a phase change, which is proportional to the velocity of flow. A phase change is only induced when the flow is parallel to the gradient, so acquisition is repeated with gradients in different directions. Phase-contrast MRA typically has a long acquisition time.

NATIVE-SPACE/TRANCE

NATIVE-SPACE is a non-contrast technique which uses an electrocardiography-triggered 3D TSE sequence to exploit the difference in arterial signal between systole and diastole. In diastole, arteries appear bright due to the slow flowing blood, whereas in systole the arteries appear dark due to fast flowing blood. Subtracting the two images removes background and venous signal, leaving only

arterial signal. This technique is often used to image peripheral arteries.

NATIVE-TrueFISP/B-TRANCE

NATIVE-TrueFISP/b-TRANCE is a non-contrast technique which uses a 3D GRE sequence to achieve bright inflowing arterial blood. This is combined with an inversion pulse with a TI set to null signal from static tissue. This technique is often used to image renal arteries.

MR Spectroscopy (MRS)

Protons have a different resonant frequency depending on their chemical environment (chemical shift). By taking a Fourier transform of the FID, a spectrum is produced showing the different frequencies present. Each peak in the spectrum relates to a specific chemical environment.

The large water peak is suppressed using multiple RF saturation pulses tuned to the resonant frequency of water. This allows the much smaller metabolite peaks to be detected. For instance in neuroimaging it is common to see peaks for N-acetyl aspartate, creatine and choline.

A very homogenous magnetic field is required to distinguish between the small differences in chemical environments of protons. Shimming is used to correct magnetic-field inhomogeneities for each patient at the start of the scan. A good shim will produce narrow and distinct peaks. A poor shim will produce broad and difficult to distinguish peaks. Spectroscopy is generally performed at higher field strengths due to a better spectral resolution and higher SNR.

The area under the peak gives the relative number of protons and can be used to compare the relative concentrations of different metabolites. To improve SNR, a long TR (>2000 ms) and short TE (30 ms) are usually utilised.

Some peaks are split into multiple peaks. An example of this is lactate, which splits into a doublet. Lactate protons become in and out of phase due to J-coupling; therefore, when TE = 30 ms, the peak is positive, as the spins are in phase, and when TE = 144 ms, the peak is negative, as the spins are out of phase. This can be useful to distinguish the lactate peak from the lipid peak, which has a similar chemical shift.

Single-voxel or multivoxel spectroscopy can be performed. Point-resolved spectroscopy is the most common single-voxel method and uses three RF pulses: 90°, 180°, and 180°. During each RF pulse, a slice-selective gradient is applied and so the resulting spectrum is localised to the point where these three slices intersect.

It is also possible to perform quantitative spectroscopy using water as an internal reference. Spectroscopy is most commonly used in the head but can also be used in other areas.

Diffusion-Weighted Imaging (DWI)

Diffusion is the microscopic random movement of molecules. Diffusion is different to flow because, in diffusion, there is no net change in the average location of molecules. The amount of diffusion is measured by the diffusion coefficient, D.

Diffusion can be isotropic (equal in all directions) or restricted in one or more directions (Fig. 6.32).

Restricted diffusion can indicate pathology. Cancerous tissues show increased cellularity which can cause restricted diffusion. In ischaemic stroke, cytotoxic oedema results in restricted diffusion.

DWI utilises a SE sequence with two large equal gradients applied either side of the $180°$ pulse. The first gradient causes dephasing of spins. The second gradient will rephase spins only if they are in the same position. For spins that have diffused, signal is only partially rephased.

In DWI, tissues with mobile molecules appear dark and tissues where diffusion is restricted appear bright.

Images are acquired with at least two different diffusion weightings, also known as 'b-values'. Higher b-values show a greater dependence on diffusion. The b-value is determined by the gradient strength, duration, and the spacing between the two gradient pulses.

Different b-value images can be combined to form an apparent diffusion coefficient (ADC) map. Only two images are required to create an ADC map; however, more b-values will increase accuracy. One low b-value image is typically acquired (this can be b = 0), but for some applications, a slightly higher b-value is preferred to avoid contributions from perfusion effects.

In ADC maps, the image contrast is flipped. Free diffusion appears bright and restricted diffusion appears dark.

TABLE 6.4   Appearance of Different Tissues on DWI and ADC Images

	DWI	ADC
Restricted diffusion	Bright	Dark
Increased diffusion	Dark	Bright
T_2-shine-through	Bright	Bright

ADC, apparent diffusion coefficient; DWI, diffusion-weighted imaging.

DWI is not just dependent on the diffusion coefficient of tissue but is also partly T_2-weighted. If a tissue has a very long T_2 value, it can appear bright on DWI and mimic restricted diffusion. This is known as 'T_2 shine-through'. The ADC map removes the T_2 dependence and so can be used to distinguish true restricted diffusion from T_2 shine-through (Table 6.4).

Higher b-value images suffer from low SNR. It is possible to create higher b-value images from lower b-value data by extrapolation.

Diffusion Tensor Imaging (DTI)

When diffusion is restricted in a particular direction, this is referred to as anisotropic.

DTI uses the same principles as DWI but applies the diffusion gradients in many more directions. Only diffusion occurring parallel to the applied gradient will result in signal loss; by applying many gradients, preferred diffusion direction information can be obtained.

DTI can be used to map out the white matter tracts in brain tissue, as diffusion occurs preferentially along the white matter bundles. This can be used in pre-surgical planning.

Perfusion Imaging

There are several different sequences which are used to create perfusion maps.

Dynamic Susceptibility Contrast (DSC)

DSC is commonly used in the brain. A gadolinium bolus is injected, and rapid T_2w or T_2*w images are acquired pre-contrast and throughout the first pass of the bolus. Gadolinium causes the blood to show a reduced signal. The change in signal can be used to produce maps such as time to peak (TTP), mean transit time (MTT), cerebral blood volume (CBV), and cerebral blood flow (CBF).

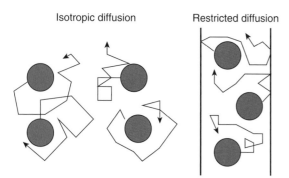

Isotropic diffusion   Restricted diffusion

Fig. 6.32 (A) Isotropic diffusion. (B) Restricted diffusion.

Dynamic Contrast-Enhanced (DCE)

DCE is used in areas such as liver, prostate, breast, and heart. A gadolinium bolus is injected, and rapid T_1w images are acquired pre-contrast, throughout the first pass of the bolus, and at several delay times. Gadolinium causes the T_1 to decrease, so areas where gadolinium accumulates will see signal enhancement. Different patterns of contrast uptake and washout relate to different pathologies.

Arterial Spin Labelling (ASL)

One example of ASL is to apply a 180° RF labelling pulse to a volume outside of the slice of interest, which acts to label the blood. Images are acquired when the labelled blood has moved into the slice of interest. Imaging is repeated without the labelling pulse. The labelled image is subtracted from the control image. The difference is proportional to the blood flow. ASL is a non-contrast technique and so is suitable for patients where the use of gadolinium is not recommended. However, ASL suffers from low SNR, which means acquisition time tends to be long to achieve an acceptable image quality.

Susceptibility-Weighted Imaging (SWI)

In standard imaging, only the magnitude of the MR signal is utilised. In SWI, the phase data is used to provide additional information on tissues with different susceptibilities. Most commonly used in the brain, SWI is good for demonstrating paramagnetic or diamagnetic materials such as calcium, ferritin, deoxyhaemoglobin (a sign of acute haemorrhage), and haemosiderin (a sign of chronic haemorrhage). SWI can be used instead of T_2^*w GRE sequences in some areas as it shows similar information with a greater sensitivity.

Functional MRI (fMRI)

Oxyhaemoglobin is diamagnetic (weakly opposes B_0), whereas deoxyhaemoglobin is paramagnetic (weakly enhances B_0). Blood oxygenation level-dependent (BOLD) imaging is used in fMRI studies and consists of a series of rapid T_2^*w sequences acquired whilst the patient is at rest and again when performing a task. fMRI studies are most commonly used in the brain to look at areas which receive an increased supply of oxygenated blood when a task is performed. The BOLD signal is small, but increases with B_0, so fMRI is preferentially performed at high field strength. The images are typically processed and then overlaid on anatomical images.

Qualitative vs Quantitative MRI

Almost all clinical MRI use qualitative images, meaning that images are weighted with different contrasts and then visually interpreted. Quantitative techniques can be used to measure and display tissue parameters. These techniques have the potential to improve objectivity but are much more difficult to implement. The range of parameters that can be mapped include T_1, T_2, T_2^*, diffusion, perfusion, fat, water, and iron fraction and tissue stiffness.[9] It can be difficult to achieve accurate, reproducible quantitative maps, and a robust QA program must be in place if quantitative maps are to be used clinically.

REFERENCES

1. Medicines and Healthcare Regulatory Agency. *Safety Guidelines for Magnetic Resonance Imaging Equipment in Clinical Use*; 2021. Version 4.3 [Online]. Available at: https://www.gov.uk/government/publications/safety-guidelines-for-magnetic-resonance-imaging-equipment-in-clinical-use (Accessed on: 31 May 2022).
2. Delfino JG, others. MRI-related FA adverse event reports: a 10-yr review. *Med Phys*. 2019;46:5562–5571.
3. Patient death illustrates the importance of adhering to safety precautions in magnetic resonance environments. *Healthc Hazard Manage Monit 15*. 2001;1–3.
4. Klucznik RP, others. Placement of a ferromagnetic intracerebral aneurysm clip in a magnetic field with a fatal outcome. *Radiology*. 1993;187:855–856.
5. Haik J, others. MRI induced fourth-degree burn in an extremity, leading to amputation. *Burns*. 2009;35:294–296.
6. The Royal College of Radiologists. *Guidance on Gadolinium-Based Contrast Agent Administration to Adult Patients*. London, UK: Royal College of Radiologists; 2019.
7. Kanda T, others. High signal intensity in the dentate nucleus and globus pallidus on unenhanced T1-weighted MR images: relationship with increasing cumulative dose of a gadolinium-based contrast material. *Radiology*. 2014;270:834–841.
8. Press statement from European Medicines Agency. *PRAC Confirms Restrictions on the Use of Linear Gadolinium Agents*; 2017 [Online]. Available at: https://www.ema.europa.eu/en/documents/referral/gadolinium-article-31-referral-prac-confirms-restrictions-use-linear-gadolinium-agents_en.pdf (Accessed: 31 May 2022).

9. McRobbie D, Moore E, Graves M, Prince M. *MRI From Picture to Proton*. 3rd ed. Cambridge, UK: Cambridge University Press; 2017.

10. Ridgway JP. Cardiovascular magnetic resonance physics for clinicians: part I. *J Cardiovasc Magn Reson*. 2010;12:71.

11. Biglands JD, Radjenovic A, Ridgway JP. Cardiovascular magnetic resonance physics for clinicians: part II. *J Cardiovasc Magn Reson*. 2012;14(1):66.

12. Institute of Physics and Engineering in Medicine. *Report 112 Quality Control and Artefacts in Magnetic Resonance Imaging*. X ed. York, UK: Institute of Physics and Engineering in Medicine; 2017.

13. Morelli JN, others. An image-based approach to understanding the physics of MR artifacts. *Radiographics*. 2011;31:849–866.

14. Elster AD. *Questions and Answers in MRI*; 2021. Available at: https://www.MRIquestions.com [Online]. (Accessed on: 1 June 2021).

FURTHER READING

Medicines and Healthcare Regulatory Agency. *Safety Guidelines for Magnetic Resonance Imaging Equipment in Clinical Use*; 2021. Version 4.3 [Online] Available at: https://www.gov.uk/government/publications/safety-guidelines-for-magnetic-resonance-imaging-equipment-in-clinical-use (Accessed on: 31 May 2022).

McRobbie D, Moore E, Graves M, Prince M. *MRI From Picture to Proton*. 3rd ed. Cambridge, UK: Cambridge University Press; 2017.

Elster AD. *Questions and Answers in MRI*; 2021. Available at: https://www.MRIquestions.com [Online]. (Accessed on: 1 June 2021).

7

Ultrasound Imaging

INTRODUCTION

Sound is the physical vibration of particles in a medium — *not* electromagnetic (EM) radiation (e.g., light and X-rays). Like light (but unlike X-rays and gamma rays), sound can be reflected, refracted, and focussed. Unlike electromagnetic waves, sound requires a medium in which to travel.

Ultrasound is sound with a frequency above the human audible range (>20 kHz). Audible sound spreads through a room, whereas the short wavelengths of ultrasound allow it to be directed into a beam. Advantages of ultrasound over X-ray imaging include superior soft tissue contrast, and safety — for example in obstetric imaging — due to perceived comparatively insignificant hazards.

Longitudinal compression waves travel in the direction of particle movement (see Fig. 7.1). Particles moving closer together result in increased pressure (compression) and particles moving apart result in reduced pressure (rarefaction). Normal pressure at 1 atm is 101 kPa. Longitudinal waves are those used in standard ultrasound imaging. Transverse shear waves travel in the direction perpendicular

to particle motion (Fig. 7.2). This type of wave can be used in shear wave elastography.

PHYSICAL PROPERTIES OF ULTRASOUND

The **frequency** (*f*) of a sound wave is how many times per second the compression phase passes any single point in the medium, measured in megahertz (MHz). The **period** (*T*) of a wave is the *time* between successive compressions (or rarefactions) *at a single position in the medium* (Fig. 7.1A).

$$T = \frac{1}{f}$$

The **wavelength** (*λ*) of a wave is the *distance* between successive compressions (or rarefactions) *at a single point in time* (Fig. 7.1B). The **speed of sound** (*c*) depends on the medium through which it travels. In tissue, ultrasound behaves as in a fluid, so the speed of sound

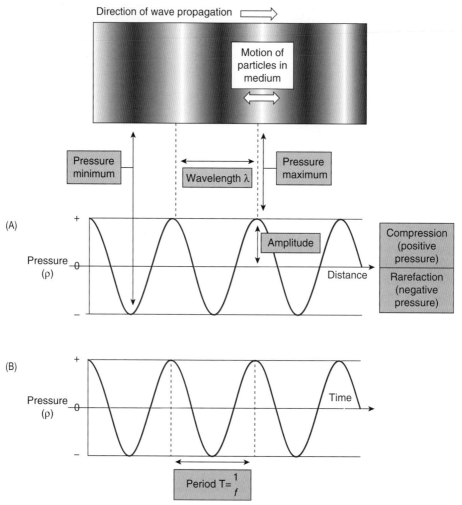

(A)

Fig. 7.1 Propagation of a longitudinal pressure wave and graphs of the sinusoidal continuous waves showing excess pressure (A) versus distance and (B) versus time.

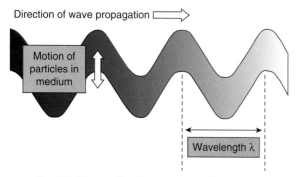

Fig. 7.2 Propagation of a transverse shear wave.

$$c = \sqrt{\frac{B}{\rho}}$$

Hence, sound speed increases with the stiffness and decreases with the density of the medium. It also increases with temperature. Table 7.1 shows the density and speed of sound in various media. Air has a much lower density, but is much more compressible than water or tissue, hence the low velocity.

For practical purposes, sound travels through a homogeneous medium at a constant speed c that is independent of frequency and wavelength:

$$c = f\lambda$$

depends on the stiffness (adiabatic elastic bulk modulus, B) and density (ρ):

TABLE 7.1   Properties of Ultrasound in Various Media

Material	Speed (c) (m/s)	Density (ρ) (kg/m³)
Air	330	1.29
Average soft tissue	1540[a]	1000
Typical bone	3200	1650
Lead zirconate titanate (PZT)	4000	7500

[a]Range of speed: 1300–1800 m/s

TABLE 7.2   Acoustic Impedances of Various Media

Tissue	Acoustic Impedance (Z) (kg/m²s)
Air	430
Muscle	1.70×10^6
Liver	1.64×10^6
Spleen	1.63×10^6
Kidney	1.62×10^6
Average soft tissue	1.5×10^6
Fat	1.38×10^6
Typical bone	5.3×10^6
Lead zirconate titanate (PZT)	30×10^6

The intensity of ultrasound, measured in watts per square millimetre (W/mm²), is proportional to the square of the wave amplitude (Fig. 7.1A) and is under the operator's control.

Interference is the interaction that occurs when two waves cross each other (Fig. 7.3).

- Constructive interference occurs when the two waves are exactly in step (in phase) and their amplitudes add up.
- Destructive interference occurs when the two waves are out of phase. This results in a reduction in intensity. If they are equal and exactly out of phase, they completely cancel out.

Acoustic impedance (Z) describes the resistance experienced by an ultrasound beam in the medium. It depends on density (ρ) and elasticity and is, for practical purposes, independent of frequency. Acoustic impedance is measured in Rayls (kg/m²s) and can be calculated using the speed of sound in the medium:

$$Z = \rho c$$

Examples of impedance in various media are given in Table 7.2. The fraction of sound energy reflected and transmitted between two media depends on the acoustic impedance.

PIEZOELECTRIC EFFECT

Piezoelectric materials convert electrical energy into sound energy and vice versa (Fig. 7.4). These allow charge accumulation after the application of mechanical stresses. Such materials used in ultrasound include lead zirconate titanate (PZT) composite or plastic polyvinylidine difluoride (PVDF). When heated above the Curie temperature (individual for each material; e.g., 350°C for PZT), the piezoelectric properties are lost.

In an ultrasound transducer, two opposite faces are coated with electrically conducting silver. To produce an

(A)

(B)

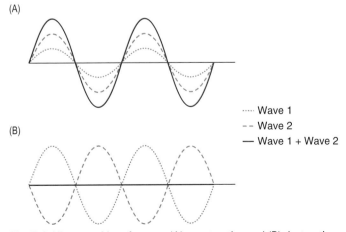

···· Wave 1
-- Wave 2
— Wave 1 + Wave 2

Fig. 7.3 Ultrasound interference: (A) constructive and (B) destructive.

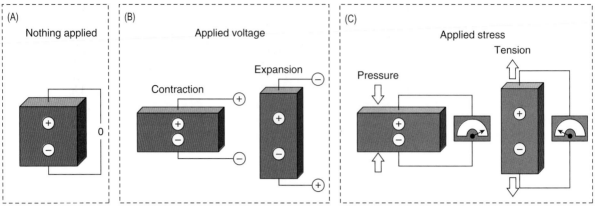

Fig. 7.4 Piezoelectric material with (A) nothing applied; (B) a voltage applied across the transducer, causing a mechanical oscillation; and (C) a stress applied, producing a voltage across the transducer.

ultrasound wave, a voltage is applied across the piezoelectric material, causing it to expand or contract (Fig. 7.4B). This effect is proportional to the voltage and reverses if the voltage is reversed. When coupled with a medium, this creates a pressure wave, which travels through the medium.

To detect ultrasound: the incoming pressure wave creates a voltage across the transducer (Fig. 7.4C), which can be detected. Hence, the transducer converts sound energy to electrical energy and vice versa, so acting as a both a transmitter and receiver.

WAVE TYPES

Continuous wave (CW)

Applying an alternating current (AC) voltage causes continuous expansion and contraction at same frequency. Conversely, applying an alternating pressure causes an alternating voltage at the same frequency. This wave takes a sinusoidal form (Fig. 7.1A and B).

Pulsed wave (PW)

Applying a direct current (DC) voltage causes a short period of expansion and compression, due to the elasticity of the medium. After the DC 'hit', the transducer continues to vibrate, but loses energy exponentially (in the form of sound), producing a short pulse of ultrasound (Fig. 7.5). This type of pulse is used in ultrasound imaging. Pulse length can be defined in terms of time or distance. The length of an imaging pulse is typically up to 3 wavelengths or periods. For example, at 3 MHz:

$$Pulse\ Length\ (distance) = 3\lambda = 3 \times \frac{c}{f}$$

$$= 3 \times \frac{1540}{3 \times 10^6} = 1.5\ mm$$

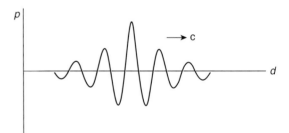

Fig. 7.5 Excess pressure versus distance for a pulsed wave.

$$Pulse\ Length\ (time) = 3T = 3 \times \frac{\lambda}{c}$$

$$= 3 \times \frac{1.5 \times 10^{-3}}{1540} = 1\ \mu s$$

As speed is assumed to be the same in tissue, time and distance can effectively be interchanged.

Damping, when applied to an ultrasound transducer, causes loss (decay) of energy and shortens the pulse length (Fig. 7.6). **Ringing** is the continuation of pulse vibrations and occurs when there is little or no damping.

Frequency spectrum

In CW, a single frequency (e.g., a pure tone) is emitted. The frequency spectrum, which plots relative intensity against frequency, is a single line A in Fig. 7.7. In PW, the pulse contains a range of frequencies: a continuous spectrum of sine waves that combine to produce the pulse B or C is shown in Fig. 7.7.

Bandwidth describes the range of frequencies contained in a pulse and is defined as the full width at half maximum of the frequency spectrum. The shorter the pulse, the larger the bandwidth.

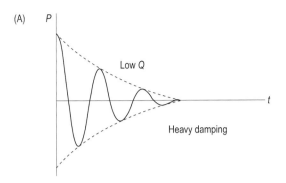

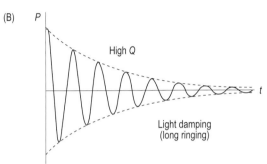

Fig. 7.6 Damping: (A) heavy and (B) light.

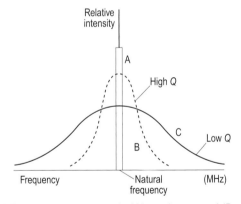

Fig. 7.7 Frequency spectrum in (A) continuous and (B and C) pulsed modes

SINGLE-TRANSDUCER PROBE

Fig. 7.8 shows the basic components of a single-transducer ultrasound probe. The piezoelectric element is used to transmit and receive the ultrasound.

Resonant (natural) frequency

In Fig. 7.9, the front face of the transducer emits sound both forwards and backwards. The back wave B is reflected at the back face. By the time it meets the front wave F, it has travelled an extra distance of twice the crystal thickness: 2t. If, as in the diagram, this distance is equal to one

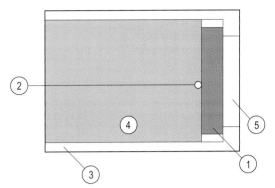

Fig. 7.8 Section through a single-transducer probe. 1, Piezoelectric element; 2, insulated wire; 3, earthed metal case; 4, backing block; 5, lens.

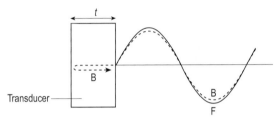

Fig. 7.9 Resonance. B and F are the backward and forward-travelling waves, respectively. t is the transducer crystal thickness.

wavelength. F and B are perfectly in phase, resulting in maximum constructive interference. The corresponding frequency is the resonant frequency and therefore depends on t and the speed of sound in the crystal. If using DC, the transducer will naturally vibrate at the resonant frequency, with a wavelength of:

$$\lambda = 2t$$

For example: for a 4 MHz transducer in PZT crystal, the thickness would be:

$$\frac{1}{2}\lambda = \frac{1}{2} \times \frac{c}{f} = \frac{1}{2} \times \frac{4000}{4 \times 10^6} \approx 0.5 \text{ mm}$$

Hence, a thicker crystal resonates at a lower frequency, producing a longer wavelength.

In general, a range of thicknesses can be used when driven with AC at a chosen resonant frequency (where n is any integer):

$$\lambda = 2n \times crystal\ thickness$$

The transducer is most sensitive when operating at the resonant frequency. Most modern transducers operate across a bandwidth (e.g., 1–5 MHz). To use a frequency outside this range, one would have to change transducer.

Mechanical coefficient (Q factor) describes the bandwidth of frequencies produced by a given crystal (Fig. 7.7), defined by the centre frequency (f_0) and the bandwidth (Δf):

$$Q = \frac{f_0}{\Delta f}$$

A high Q transducer produces a pure tone and only responds to a single frequency, as in CW. A low Q transducer has a short ring-down time, produces short pulses, and produces and responds to a wide range of frequencies, as in PW.

Electrodes

The voltage is applied to the crystal between an insulated wire and earthed metal case.

Backing Block

The transducer is mounted onto a block of material such as tungsten powder in epoxy resin. This is *matched* to the transducer material to enable transmission backwards and is used to absorb the ultrasound and damp the vibration, like placing a hand on a vibrating drum skin, enabling shorter pulses. The disadvantages of damping are reduction in output and reduced Q factor. CW ultrasound transducers are therefore typically air-backed.

Lens

A layer of material (the lens) such as plastic or silicone is affixed to the front face of the transducer, performing several functions:
- Protects the surface of the element from damage
- Insulates the patient from the applied voltage
- Focuses the beam (like an optical lens)
- Improves transmission into the patient from the transducer by acoustic 'matching'

ULTRASOUND BEAM

If the element diameter (aperture size) D is smaller than one wavelength (e.g., 0.5 mm), sound will spread equally in all directions as spherical waves and would have no directional properties (Fig. 7.10A).

If D is much larger, sound is projected forwards, effectively as a plane wave. As in Fig. 7.10B, the transducer can be thought of as several mini-transducers. For every crest that reaches any point B outside the beam from one mini-transducer, a trough arrives from another, causing destructive interference and in general cancelling out. Within the beam, the separate sound waves that reach point A within the beam are more or less on phase, so constructively interfere and reinforce. As a result, most of the energy is confined within an ultrasound beam of width D.

Focus: The intensity of the beam is naturally concentrated at a defined depth, known as the beam focus. At this depth, the amplitude of the beam is increased and the width of the beam at its narrowest. The behaviour of the ultrasound beam changes with depth and can be divided into two portions, divided by the beam's natural focus:

The **near field (Fresnel region)** extends from the transducer face and remains nearly parallel up to the focus. The near field length is calculated by:

$$N = \frac{\left(D/2\right)^2}{\lambda}$$

Hence, N is proportional to fD^2.

The **far field (Fraunhofer region)** extends beyond the focus, where the interference effect is lost, and the beam diverges. The angle of divergence is calculated by:

$$\sin \theta = 1.2 \frac{\lambda}{D}$$

Hence, increasing frequency or aperture size reduces far field divergence.

For example: at 3.5 MHz with aperture size $D = 12$ mm:

$$N = \frac{\left(D/2\right)^2}{\lambda} = \frac{\left(6 \times 10^{-3}\right)^2}{4.4 \times 10^{-4}} = 82 \text{ mm}$$

$$\theta = \sin^{-1}\left(1.2 \frac{4.4 \times 10^{-4}}{12 \times 10^{-3}}\right) = \sin^{-1}(0.044) = 2.5°$$

BEHAVIOUR OF A BEAM AT INTERFACES

If a beam strikes the boundary between two media (transducer-skin, tissue-bone, tissue-air etc.), some energy is reflected as an 'echo' and some is transmitted through the interface.

The portion of the beam that is reflected towards the transducer is detected and contributes to the image. The portion that is transmitted continues through the tissue and is either detected due to subsequent reflections or is lost due to attenuation.

Specular reflection

This occurs if:
- The beam strikes a large, smooth interface that is *larger than the wavelength*
- The acoustic impedance of the tissues on either side of the interface are non-equal ($Z_1 \neq Z_2$)

It is analogous to light reflecting off a mirror. As with light, the angle of reflection is equal to the angle of

(A)

(B)

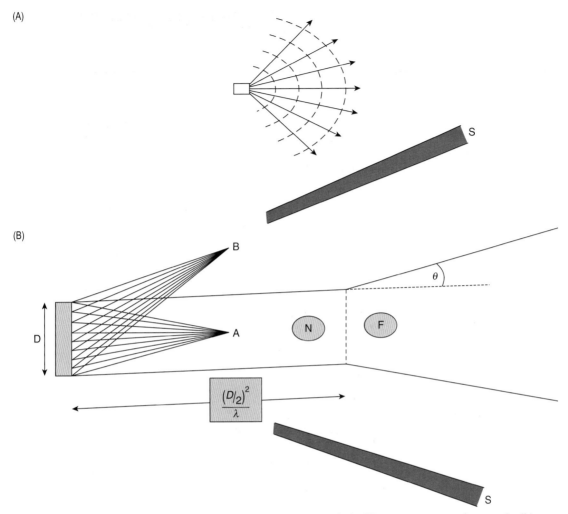

Fig. 7.10 Pattern of sound emitted by (A) a very small aperture: dashed lines represent wavefronts and solid lines show direction of propagation; and (B) a larger aperture with near (N) and far (F) fields.

incidence (Fig. 7.11A). If the ultrasound beam is at or close to right angles to the interface, the fraction of the beam that is reflected (*R*) can be calculated as:

$$R = \frac{(Z_1 - Z_2)^2}{(Z_1 + Z_2)^2}$$

Hence, the greater the difference in *Z*, the greater the fraction *R* reflected (Table 7.3).

Small variations in soft tissues result in small fractions of reflection, e.g., nearly 1% at a kidney-fat interface. This enables visualisation of internal anatomical structures such as organ boundaries.

For example: for a bone/muscle interface, the reflected fraction is:

$$R = \frac{(5.3 - 1.7)^2}{(5.3 + 1.7)^2} \approx 30\%$$

Hence, approximately 70% is transmitted through the interface. In general, it is not possible to image through bone due in part to reflection, but also to high levels of absorption.

In air, *Z* is negligible, resulting in total reflection and no transmission. Anatomy that is behind gas-filled organs cannot be imaged. The bowel wall can therefore be imaged,

(A)

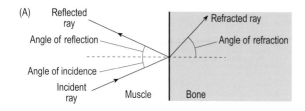

(B)

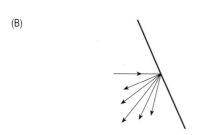

(C)

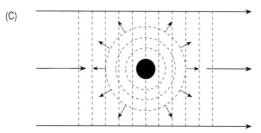

Fig. 7.11 (A) Specular reflection, transmission, and refraction. The angle of reflection is equal to the angle of incidence and the angle of refraction is determined by Snell's law. (B) Diffuse reflection and (C) scattering.

but not the lumen itself. Sound cannot travel from the transducer into the tissue if air is trapped between the transducer face and the skin. Hence, acoustic coupling gel is used, and bubbles must be avoided.

Acoustic matching

If $Z_1 = Z_2$:

$$R = 0$$

$$\text{therefore } (1 - R) = 1$$

Hence, 100% of the energy is transmitted. This means that the media are *acoustically matched*, as should be the case for the transducer and backing block.

Matching layer. PZT crystal has a very high Z (Table 7.1), so if transmitting directly into tissue, most of the ultrasound is reflected:

TABLE 7.3   Typical Reflection Factors

Interface	Reflected Fraction (%)
Gas-tissue	99.9
Soft tissue – lead zirconate titanate	80
Bone-muscle	30
Plastic–soft tissue	10
Fat-muscle	1
Blood-muscle	0.1
Liver-muscle	0.01

$$R = \frac{(30 - 1.5)^2}{(30 + 1.5)^2} \approx 80\%$$

To allow greater transmission, a matching layer is used (often in the form of the lens), with an intermediate acoustic impedance Z_2 chosen such that:

$$Z_2 = \sqrt{Z_1 Z_3}$$

For the above example:

$$Z_2 = \sqrt{30 \times 1.5} = 6.7$$

The thickness of the matching layer also affects transmission, due to interference.

Diffuse reflection

This is the same effect as that seen with light and frosted glass. It occurs if the beam strikes a rough interface with *undulations approximately equal to 1 wavelength*. The incident beam is reflected over a range of angles (Fig. 7.11B). This spread is greater on rougher surfaces and for shorter wavelengths. When this happens at multiple surfaces, some reflections may return to the transducer even if they did not strike an interface at right angles. Diffuse reflections contribute to most of the generated ultrasound image.

(Rayleigh-like) scatter

This occurs if the beam encounters a structure that is *much smaller than the wavelength* (e.g., red blood corpuscle, diameter 10 µm, or tissue parenchyma). The beam is scattered in all directions and produces an interference pattern that does not directly represent but is related to the tissue structure, as well as the wavelength (Fig. 7.11C). This enables visualisation and characterisation of the interior of tissues such as placenta, liver, pancreas, spleen, and kidney. The signal received from scatter is usually 1%–10% as strong as from organ boundaries.

Refraction

This occurs at an interface if the speeds of sound of the tissues on either side of the interface are non-equal ($c_1 \neq c_2$). The portion of the beam that is transmitted will continue along an altered angle, θ_2 (Fig. 7.11A), calculated using Snell's law:

$$\frac{\sin \theta_1}{\sin \theta_2} = \frac{c_1}{c_2}$$

ATTENUATION

When travelling through a medium, sound energy is lost to the surrounding medium. This happens due to:

- **Absorption** — As the ultrasound travels through tissue, processes such as friction and viscous forces convert the mechanical energy into heat energy, which is absorbed by the tissue. In soft tissue, absorption is approximately proportional to frequency, so higher frequencies are more readily absorbed.
- **Scattering** and **reflection** from interfaces, removing energy from the forward-travelling beam.

Attenuation is quantified using the ratio of the power or intensity of the incident and transmitted beam — P_i and P_t (W) or I_i and I_t (W/m^2 or W m^{-2}) — over a given distance x. As ratio values can vary widely, it is simpler to represent these on a logarithmic (rather than linear) scale in decibels (dB).

$$Decibels = 10 \log_{10}(Power\ or\ Intensity\ Ratio)$$

Note that decibels are additive. Positive values show amplification and negative values attenuation. The attenuation of a medium is quantified by the attenuation coefficient as follows:

$$Attenuation\ Coefficient = -\frac{1}{x} 10 \log_{10}\left(\frac{I_t}{I_i}\right) dB\ cm^{-1}$$

Typical values are given in Table 7.4.

There is little attenuation in water, so a full bladder can allow the ultrasound to reach deeper structures. Bone and air attenuate much more, so it is very difficult to image through ribs and bowel gas.

The **half-value layer** is the thickness of tissue that reduces the intensity to half. This corresponds to a change of: $\log_{10}\left(\frac{1}{2}\right) = -3$ dB. For example: the half-value layer at 1 MHz in average tissue (0.7 dB/cm) would be:

$$HVL = -\frac{\log_{10}\left(\frac{1}{2}\right)}{0.7} = 4.3\ cm$$

At a certain depth, the intensity of the beam has reduced so much that it is no longer useful. This depth of penetration is poorer at higher frequencies, as attenuation is greater. Roughly, penetration (cm) $= {}^{40}/_f$.

A-MODE (AMPLITUDE MODE)

A-mode is the simplest form of ultrasound imaging, producing a simple representation of the depth of tissue interfaces along a single line (Fig. 7.12). This has now been largely replaced by B-mode, but has been used for examining the eye, identifying midline displacement in the brain, and identifying cysts in the breast.

1. The probe face is held against the patient and an ultrasound pulse is transmitted into the tissue.
2. This pulse takes a time t to reach interface a.
3. Some of the energy is reflected back along the path towards the transducer, taking an additional time t to reach the transducer (i.e., a total round-trip time of $2t$).

TABLE 7.4 **Typical Tissue Attenuation Values (Approximate)**				
		HALF-VALUE LAYER (CM)		
Tissue Type	**Attenuation (dB/cm at 1 MHz)**	**1 MHz**	**2 MHz**	**5 MHz**
Water	0.0022	1360	340	54
Blood	0.18	17	8.5	3
Average Tissue	0.7	4.3	2.1	0.9
Bone	15	0.2	0.1	0.04
Lung	40	0.08	0.04	0.02

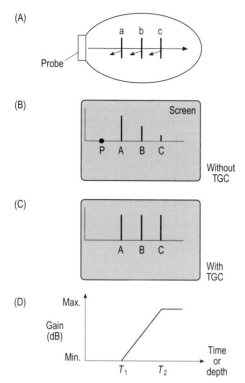

Fig. 7.12 A-mode: (A) section through transducer and patient, (B) trace on screen without time gain control, (C) trace on screen using time gain control, and (D) variation of gain with depth. *TGC*, time gain compensation.

4. The transducer acts as a receiver and converts the sound energy into an electrical pulse.
   The depth of the interface can be calculated using:

$$depth_a = c \times t_a$$

   where c is the assumed speed of sound and $t =$ half the time between transmission and reception.

5. This signal is amplified and a short vertical trace ('blip') is produced on the screen at the calculated depth. The other interfaces b and c then produce corresponding blips.

6. Pulses are transmitted and received at regular intervals to refresh the image.

B-MODE (BRIGHTNESS MODE)

Rather than imaging a one-dimensional line through the patient, B-mode allows imaging of a two-dimensional slice (similar to a single slice in computed tomography).

As in A-mode, the transducer is pulsed at regular intervals, however in B-mode, the ultrasound beam is scanned sequentially across a two-dimensional section, either:

- Linearly to produce a rectangular image
- Rotationally to produce a sector image

Fig. 7.13 shows the scan lines travelled by each pulse to produce the image. Only boundaries approximately perpendicular to the scan lines will be imaged.

The returning echo pulses are displayed as bright pixels on the screen. The image is built up as a series of vertical lines on the screen, corresponding to each ultrasound beam in the sequence, and displayed on the monitor screen in a matrix of pixels (e.g., 512 × 512 or 1074 × 768), corresponding to the matrix of voxels in the scanned anatomy:

- The lateral (horizontal) pixel position is determined by the position of the beam relative to the patient surface, or the angle of the beam.
- The axial (vertical) pixel position is determined by the depth calculated from the round-trip time.
- The brightness of the pixel is determined by the strength of the received signal. As the signal strength depends on the strength of reflection from the corresponding interface, this enables tissue differentiation based on the pixel brightness.
- A real-time image is displayed on the monitor screen in a matrix of pixels, corresponding to the matrix of voxels in the body.

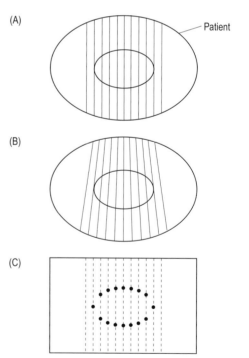

Fig. 7.13 B-mode: (A) linear scan, (B) sector scan, and (C) the monitor screen.

TABLE 7.5 Methods of Producing a Two-Dimensional Image

Scan Method	Pros	Cons	Applications
Mechanical Sector Scanning	• Cheap • Focussed beam allows better resolution than phased array	• Moving parts • Probes can be cumbersome	• Transrectal imaging • 4D imaging
Electronic Linear or Curvilinear Array	• Wide field throughout the image • Good image quality	• Wide probe face requires a large area of patient contact • Curvilinear line density reduced with depth due to beam divergence	• Flat linear probes: superficial vessels and nerves, thyroid • Curvilinear probes: abdomen, liver, obstetrics and gynaecology
Electronic Steered/Phased Array	• Smaller probe face so requires a smaller acoustic window • Smaller probe is easier to manipulate • Wider field at depth	• Narrower field at the surface • Generally lower image quality	• Used to image the heart through intercostal spaces or the infant brain through the fontanel • Also used for intracavity probes, including endoscopic probes for imaging the heart

Ultrasound images can be produced in a variety of ways depending on the clinical applications and each has its own advantages and disadvantages (Table 7.5).

REAL-TIME IMAGING

In most B-mode scanners, these two-dimensional images are produced continuously in a rapid succession of frames so that moving structures can effectively be viewed in real-time. Real-time imaging also allows large volumes to be scanned in a short amount of time. Various aspects of the real-time image can be influenced directly or indirectly by the user either by choice of transducer, or of scanner settings.

Scan line density:

The image is divided into several vertical lines with a width defined by the distance between each beam. The greater the number of lines per unit distance, or line density, the better the lateral resolution.

Pulse repetition frequency (PRF):

The rate at which pulses are transmitted along one line, measured in Hz (pulses per second):

$$PRF = \frac{1}{time\ between\ pulses}$$

Depth of view:

To image structures at depth, a pulse must have time to make the full round trip to and from the deepest structure, so:

$$depth\ of\ view = 0.5 \times \frac{c}{PRF}$$

Frame rate:

To produce a two-dimensional frame, all lines in the frame must be produced sequentially, before starting again to produce the next frame. The frame rate is the number of frames produced each second (Hz).

$$frame\ rate = \frac{PRF}{lines\ per\ frame}$$

Hence, frame rate can be increased by increasing PRF or reducing line density.

For example: for an image with 100 lines, to achieve a frame rate of 30 Hz would require:

$$PRF = frame\ rate \times lines\ per\ frame = 30 \times 100$$
$$= 3\ kHz$$

To successfully image moving structures, a sufficiently high frame rate is required. If the frame rate is too low, this can result in image 'lag' and blurring, particularly as the probe is moved across the patient.

It is therefore not possible to achieve a high frame rate, high line density, and image at a large depth, and these aspects must be balanced. Combining the above:

depth of view × number of scan lines × frame rate

= *constant*

SCAN TYPES

Two-dimensional B-mode images can be achieved in a number of ways, each with their own advantages (Table 7.5).

Mechanical (Sector) Scanning

This technique uses a transducer which is moved inside a fluid-filled outer case that is pressed against or inserted into the patient. This can be oscillated back and forth by an electric motor (Fig. 7.14), or a small group of transducer elements may be mounted onto a rotating rod (Fig. 7.15).

Electronic Scanning: Stepped Linear or Curvilinear Array

The more common technique for producing a scanned image is to use an elongated transducer that is divided up into multiple narrow transducer elements (typically at least 128) (Fig. 7.16).

As each element is very narrow, individually these would produce a poor beam for imaging, with a short near field and widely diverging far field. To mitigate this effect, elements are energised in overlapping groups in succession, (e.g., 1–6, 2–7, 3–8) so that a well-defined ultrasound beam can be scanned across a rectangular area with (say) 512 scan lines.

For this type of **linear transducer**, the size of the field of view is limited by the width of the probe (Fig. 7.17). Alternatively, in a **curvilinear transducer**, the transducer elements can be arranged on a curved surface (Fig. 7.18). As the lines of sight are perpendicular to the transducer surface, they spread out and can cover a wider field of view (Fig. 7.19).

Electronic Sector Scanner: Steered/Phased Array

This transducer has the same design as a stepped linear array, but is shorter, containing fewer elements. Instead of energising small groups of elements, a phased array uses all elements.

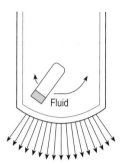

Fig. 7.14 Mechanical sector scanner with an oscillating transducer.

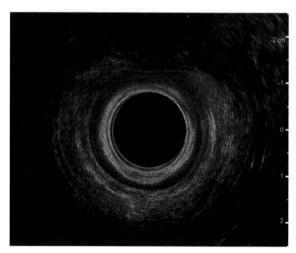

Fig. 7.15 Image of the rectum wall produced using a mechanical rotating transducer mounted inside a rod-shaped endorectal probe.

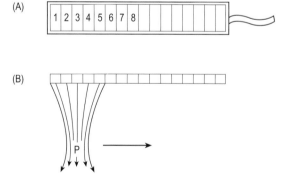

Fig. 7.16 Linear transducer array: (A) transducer face and (B) cross-section through transducer and ultrasound with electronic focussing across the scan plane.

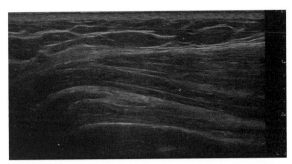

Fig. 7.17 Image of rotator cuff muscles using a linear array.

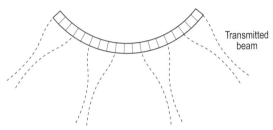

Fig. 7.18 Curvilinear array with beams spreading out perpendicular to the curved probe surface.

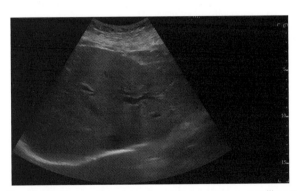

Fig. 7.19 Sector-shaped image of liver using a curvilinear transducer.

(A)

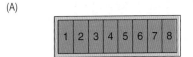

(B)

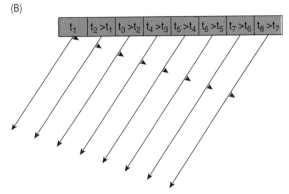

Fig. 7.20 (A) Phased array (B) timings and resulting steered beam.

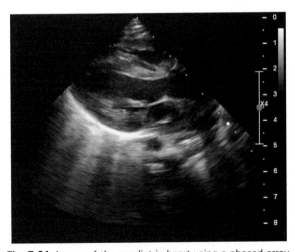

Fig. 7.21 Image of the paediatric heart using a phased array.

Steering: If energised simultaneously, the individual elements act as a single transducer with a beam directed forwards. If small delays are introduced in rapid sequence along the transducer, the pulses reinforce at an angle from the transducer face and destructively interfere in all other directions, producing a steered plane wave (Fig. 7.20). Changing the delay timing changes the angle of the beam, so this can be swept across the field of view producing a sector-shaped image (Fig. 7.21).

Intracavity Probes

To reduce the need for good penetration and to avoid the obscuring effects of bone or bowel gas, transducer arrays can be arranged on a probe that is designed for imaging intracavitarily (Table 7.6).

TABLE 7.6	Typical Types of Intracavity Probes	
Probe Type	**Application**	**Variations**
Transrectal	• Prostate • Rectum wall	• Linear array along the length • Tightly curved array at the end for a sector view • Rotating mechanical probe
Transvaginal	• Gynaecology • Obstetrics	• Tightly curved array at the end for a sector view
Endoscopic	• Cardiac (transoesophageal) • Transvascular	• Small, high-frequency phased array • Very small array with miniaturised electronics

POWER AND GAIN

The amplitude of the returning echo depends on the amplitude of the incident beam, the ratio of acoustic impedances, and the level of attenuation from interceding tissues. Hence, some interfaces may not be visualised at lower transmission amplitudes. Power and gain are two strategies for overcoming this:

Power: Increasing the output power increases the amplitude of the transmitted wave so that greater amplitude reflections are received. This also imparts more energy into the tissue, contributing to greater tissue heating.

Gain: If small signals are still detected by the transducer but not seen clearly on the image, the brightness can be increased by electrical amplification of the received signals, or increasing the overall gain. This amplifies both the 'real' received signal and any electrical noise inherent to the system.

Time gain compensation: Due to attenuation, the transmitted ultrasound energy diminishes with increasing depth, as does the returning echo, so that interfaces deeper in the body produce weaker echoes. Attenuation is compensated for by using time gain compensation (TGC), which increases the amplification of the received echoes as time increases. The aim is to render all echoes from identical interfaces the same, independent of their depth.

In A-mode, the user can alter the slope of the ramp and (retain indent) the resulting TGC curve (Fig. 7.12). In B-mode, the user has more freedom. The image is divided into more than a single range of depths and the user can adjust the level of amplification for each depth range to achieve an optimised image.

FOCUSSING

The beam width is narrowest in the near field and at the natural focus, but this can be further reduced using additional focussing. Stronger focussing leads to a shorter focal length and a narrower (and shorter) focal region, but also leads to greater beam divergence beyond the focus. Note that the focal length for a focussed beam is not necessarily the same as the length of the near field.

Physical Focussing

Physical focussing can be achieved in a few ways (Fig. 7.22):
- A curved piezoelectric element achieves a shorter focal length using greater curvature
- An annular array uses multiple elements arranged concentrically
- A plastic or silicone acoustic lens moulded to the front of the transducer (can be convex or concave, depending on material)

Electronic Focussing

In addition to physical methods, the beam can be focussed by introducing delays in when each element in a group is energised, using a similar technique to steering. This allows the user to choose the depth at which the lateral resolution of the image should be optimised.
- The outermost pair is energised first, then each adjacent pair in succession, ending with the centre (Fig. 7.23).
- The focal point, P, is defined by the depth at which the pulses arrive together and reinforce: the greater the delays, the shorter (shallower) the focal point.

Focussing improves the beam width at the focal depth but also causes greater divergence beyond the focus. This can be mitigated using multiple-zone focussing:
- For each line, multiple pulses are sent with different focal depths.
- The transducer is gated so it receives only echoes from the chosen focal depth.
- The data from each focal depth is then stitched together to produce one frame with several focal depths.

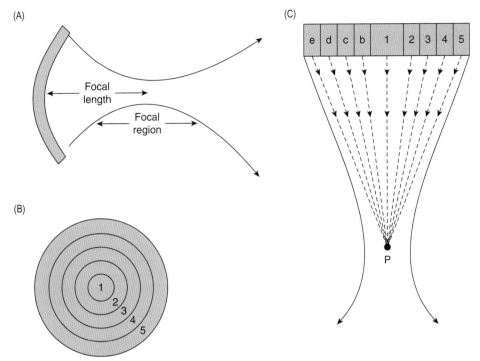

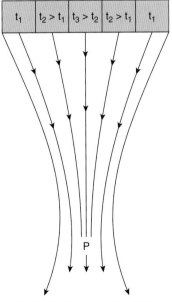

Fig. 7.22 (A) Focussed beam from a curved transducer, annular array, (B) transducer face, and (C) cross-section through the transducer and resultant focussed beam.

Fig. 7.23 Electronic focussing.

- If the focussing is done in transmission, multiple sets of pulses are required, so the frame rate reduces. Alternatively, instead of introducing delays to the transmitted beam, these can be added after reception. The result is that multiple focal depths can be created using the same transmitted beam and frame rate is maintained.

Note that this type of focussing is in only one plane: the azimuthal, or scan plane, parallel to the array. Focussing in the perpendicular or elevation plane is usually done using physical methods and this defines the slice thickness. Electronic focussing in the slice plane can be achieved using a '1.5D transducer', using multiple layers rather than a single layer of elements to improve the slice resolution.

TISSUE OPTIMISATION

In standard ultrasound imaging, the speed of sound is assumed to be 1540 m/s, when in fact in soft tissue this can range between 1300 and 1800 m/s. Fatty tissues such as breast tissue fit into the lower end of this range, so that aspects of image production such as electronic focussing timings are inaccurate, leading to reduced spatial resolution increased clutter.

The speed of sound can be corrected by the user, or **tissue optimisation** can be applied automatically by the system, through analysis and optimisation of features in the image such as spatial frequencies, which relate to spatial resolution.

M-MODE

M-mode is used to examine the position of moving structures over time.
- The B-mode image is frozen and used to direct a single beam (as in A-mode) along a line of interest, intersecting the moving surfaces as close to right angles as possible (Fig. 7.24).
- This line of echoes is displayed vertically on the screen.
- Each new line is displayed alongside the last one to show how the position changes with time horizontally across the screen.

The high temporal resolution of this technique allows quantitative analysis of fast-moving structures such as heart valves and the heart wall, which is hard to achieve with B-mode.

THREE- AND FOUR-DIMENSIONAL IMAGING

Three-dimensional images are obtained from a set of two-dimensional scans which are reconstructed to produce a volumetric image. This can be done in the following ways:
- The transducer is swept manually across the patient skin. Each frame is then stitched together. The geometric accuracy therefore depends on the skill of the operator.
- The transducer is moved mechanically within the probe. This requires a bulky probe with internal moving parts.
- A two-dimensional array is used to acquire two-dimensional images in two orthogonal planes, enabling real-time three-dimensional imaging, known as four-dimensional imaging. Many scanners will also perform post-processing such as volume and surface rendering

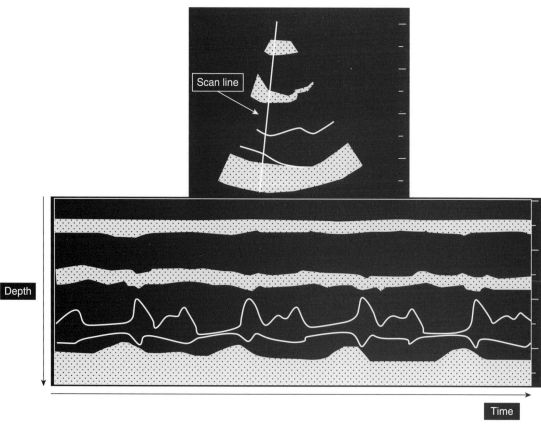

Fig. 7.24 M-mode.

to produce a three-dimensional image. This can provide useful information regarding vasculature and for foetal imaging.

IMAGE QUALITY

Signal-to-Noise Ratio (SNR)

Noise is any spurious information in the image that does not correspond to real structures in the patient. In ultrasound, noise is principally electronic noise: statistical fluctuations in the number of electrons in the very small currents measured. This appears on the image as a randomly changing 'salt-and-pepper' haze. Noise can also include any other artefacts that may obscure real anatomy, sometimes known as 'clutter'.

The **SNR** is the ratio of real signal to noise and greater SNR corresponds to better visibility of structures.

$$SNR = \frac{Real\ Signal}{Noise}$$

Contrast

The contrast between two structures is determined by the difference in the amplitudes of the reflections from each structure. High contrast makes it easy to distinguish between two structures.

Spatial Resolution

Axial (or depth) **resolution** is the ability to separate two interfaces along the same scan line. If the interfaces are too close together, the echo pulses will overlap and be recorded as a single interface (Fig. 7.25).

Axial resolution is about half the pulse length, so shorter pulses produce better axial resolution. This can be achieved by:

- Greater damping (i.e., a low Q) achieved through use of a backing layer
- Increased frequency: keeping the number of cycles in a pulse constant, a shorter wavelength will result in a shorter pulse

Lateral resolution is the ability to separate two structures side-by-side at the same depth. This depends on the beam width being narrower than the gap.

In Fig. 7.26, the width of the beam is smaller than the gap between structures A and B, so structure A is only intersected by beam 1 and structure B by beam 3. Where the beam diverges, it is wider than the gap between structures C and D, meaning that both structures are intersected by all 3 beams. Echoes from the edges of the beam are therefore misregistered in the image as having originated from the centre of the beam.

Poor lateral resolution leads to a *smearing* of small details and edges across the image. Lateral resolution in the near field is improved by using a smaller aperture and focussing.

In the focal region of the beam, axial resolution may be about one wavelength and lateral resolution about 3 times worse, being about one-third of the aperture diameter.

Slice resolution is the ability to image a structure in a narrow plane, without contribution from structures in adjacent planes. This requires a narrow beam in the slice, or elevation, plane.

Poor slice resolution leads to partial voluming, which blurs the edges of structures such as vessels and reduces

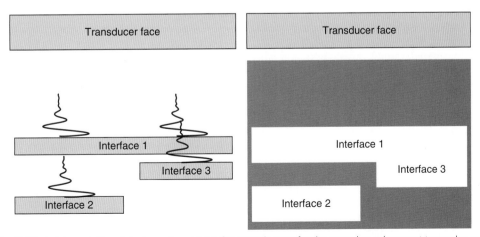

Fig. 7.25 Axial resolution. Interfaces 1 and 2 are far enough apart for the returning echoes not to overlap and allow them to be distinguished in the resulting image. Interfaces 1 and 3 are too close to each other to be distinguished separately and are merged in the resulting image.

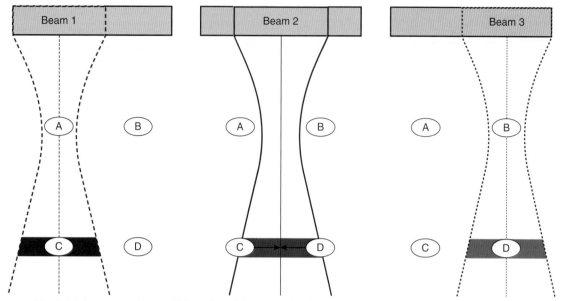

Fig. 7.26 Lateral resolution. Objects A and B are resolvable in the narrow region of beams 1 and 3, but objects C and D are not resolvable in the wider region of beam 2, with C and D merging into a single object.

visibility of small lesions. This is improved with physical focussing, or the additional electronic focussing made possible in 1.5D/3D transducers.

Resolution and Penetration

In choosing a transducer frequency for a particular investigation, it is necessary to compromise between the conflicting requirements of penetration depth (which decreases) and image resolution (which improves) as frequency is increased. Typical figures are:
- 1–8 MHz for general purpose abdominal and cardiac scanning including liver, uterus, and heart
- 5–18 MHz for thyroid, carotid, breast, testis, and other superficial tissues, and for infants
- 10–15 MHz for the eye, which is small and acoustically transparent
- Higher frequencies still may be used in imaging the skin, vessel walls, or joints

IMAGE PROCESSING

Once the raw data is acquired, the image data is processed further to optimise the image for viewing.

The smallest signal that can be detected is just greater than the noise, principally electronic noise. The detected signal dynamic range is the ratio of the maximum to the minimum signal intensity that can be detected. This is typically 70–80 dB, or 40–50 dB after TGC.

The eye can only detect around 30 grey levels, so the actual displayed dynamic range is much smaller, typically around 20–30 dB, displaying around 128–512 grey levels. This is achieved by compression: the data is divided into smaller ranges, each of which is mapped to a reduced range of grey levels (Fig. 7.27).

The amount of compression applied can be chosen depending on the requirements for the resulting image (Fig. 7.28):
- A large displayed dynamic range maps the signals to a large number of grey levels and produces a more flat, low-contrast image, in which subtle changes can be seen.
- A small displayed dynamic range maps the signals to a small number of grey levels and produces a very high-contrast image, in which high-contrast interfaces are enhanced.

The way the input signals are allocated output grey levels can be varied by altering the grey map, which can additionally enhance low-level, medium-level, or high-level signals as required. Reject control is used to filter out low-amplitude noise and scatter.

Temporal averaging (persistence):

For each point in the image, the echoes from 5–10 successive frames can be stored and combined, producing a

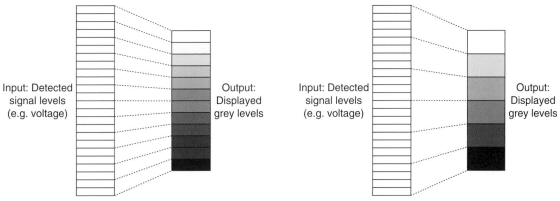

Fig. 7.27 Example of data compression, resulting in reduced dynamic range. Here, the signal range of 24 levels (e.g., voltages) are mapped to the reduced range of 12 grey levels (left) and an even lower dynamic range of 6 grey levels (right).

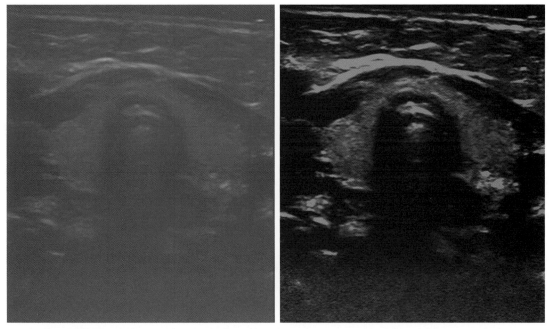

Fig. 7.28 Thyroid images showing high and low dynamic ranges on the left and right, respectively.

time-average value. Because true signals remain constant over time, these are enhanced and randomly varying noise is suppressed, producing a smoother image with increased SNR.

Spatial averaging (spatial compounding):

In this type of averaging, multiple images are produced with the beams steered over a range of angles and combined. Because true signals remain constant over time,

these are enhanced and randomly varying noise is suppressed, producing a smoother image with increased SNR.

Image enhancement:

Once the image is acquired, post-processing can be applied to either enhance or suppress certain features that aid or impede image interpretation. This can achieve effects such as speckle reduction or edge enhancement. This often takes the form of a **spatial filter**, which reassigns pixel values based on the values of surrounding pixels within the image. A smoothing filter, such as an averaging filter, assigns a pixel a value that is similar to that of the surrounding pixels, blurring image features such as speckle. A sharpening filter does the opposite, enhancing edges by increasing the weighting of pixels that contribute to those edges.

ARTEFACTS

Image formation assumes that the ultrasound:
- travels in straight lines
- speed is constant.
- attenuation is constant.
- is reflected only once from each interface.
- is transmitted in single beams perpendicular to the transducer face.

None of these assumptions hold exactly, leading to the presence of artefacts. These artefacts can lead to misdiagnosis or sometimes, when recognised, can aid in diagnosis.

Speckle:

This is produced when small structures within tissue parenchyma are too small and close together to be resolved. Instead, they scatter the ultrasound, and the scattered waves interfere, producing a textured pattern. This pattern is random and unrelated to the actual tissue texture but may be sufficiently characteristic to assist in tissue differentiation.

Reverberation:

Pairs of strongly reflecting interfaces (including transducer and skin or transducer and air — Fig. 7.29) enable multiple reflections back and forth between them before they are fully attenuated. These produce a series of delayed echoes, equally spaced, that falsely appear to be more distant structures. Comet-tail artefacts occur when these reflectors are very close, causing a tapering 'tail' of reflections distal to the reflectors (e.g., in the presence of calcifications).

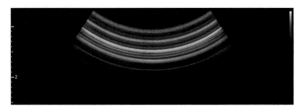

Fig. 7.29 Example of a curvilinear probe operating in air, showing multiple bands due to reverberation back and forth within the probe face.

Ring-down:

When a small gas bubble resonates, it emits ultrasound continuously, resulting in a bright track of signal throughout the scan (e.g., air in the stomach).

Mirroring:

Large, strongly reflective interfaces can act like a mirror, making structures appear displaced onto the opposite side of the interface (e.g., the diaphragm can reflect structures from the liver into the lung).

Acoustic shadowing/enhancement:

Strongly attenuating or reflecting structures reduce the intensity of distal echoes and appear to cast shadows (acoustic shadowing), e.g., bowel gas (Fig. 7.30), lung, bone, gallstones, or kidney stones. Weakly attenuating structures reduce the intensity of distal echoes less than surrounding structures and appear to produce a 'negative shadow', known as posterior acoustic enhancement (e.g., fluid-filled structures such as cysts or a filled bladder; Fig. 7.30). The scanner may try to compensate for these effects using TGC, which can be detrimental to the rest of the image, so this may need to be adjusted in the presence of acoustic shadowing or enhancement.

Distortion:

Refraction of a beam falling obliquely on an interface between tissues with very different speeds of sound displaces the beam and the images of structures beyond, causing distortion (e.g., between two surfaces of bone such as skull). Where the speed of sound is different from the assumed speed, some structures will appear shorter (e.g., lung: slower) or larger (e.g., gallstones: faster). Some scanners have variable speed of sound, such as those used in breast tissue where the sound travels slower.

Side lobes and grating lobes:

Additional, lower-intensity beams can be created which project at an angle from the central beam. These are either in the form of:
- Side lobes: caused by vibrations at the edge of the transducer element
- Grating lobes: interactions between the beams from adjacent transducer elements

If there are strong reflectors in these beams, their reflections are assumed to originate from the central beam, producing ghost structures that are displaced from their correct position.

Harmonic imaging:

As ultrasound propagates through tissue, the speed of sound varies through different tissues, so some parts of the

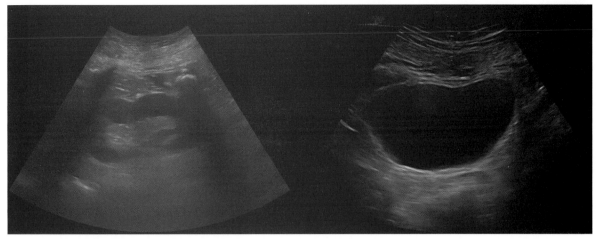

Fig. 7.30 Image of kidney showing acoustic shadowing due to bowel gas (left) and image of bladder showing postcystic enhancement (right).

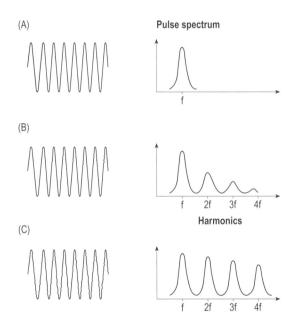

Fig. 7.31 Change in sound wave profile with different tissues at depth: (A) initial, (B) after a few centimetres of tissue, and (C) after a few more centimetres of tissue.

wave 'get ahead' or 'fall behind', distorting the wave. Hence the frequency components also change, containing not only the fundamental frequency, (first harmonic: f), but also multiples of this frequency (higher-order harmonics) (Fig. 7.31 For example: for a probe operating at 2 MHz,

the 2nd, 3rd, and 4th harmonics ($2f$, $3f$, and $4f$) would be 4, 6, and 8 MHz, respectively. This effect becomes more pronounced with depth as the wave passes through more tissue.).

In harmonic imaging, the fundamental frequency (1st harmonic) is transmitted, and both the fundamental and higher-order harmonics are reflected back to the transducer. The 2nd harmonic can produce ultrasound of a sufficient magnitude to be useful. This is separated from the fundamental to produce an image of the harmonic only. There are a variety of methods to separate the 2nd harmonic.

Band filtering: In band filtering (Fig. 7.32A), the fundamental frequency is removed using a low-pass filter. To use this technique, both the fundamental and harmonic frequencies must be contained within the probe bandwidth, but to be separable they cannot overlap, so a longer pulse is needed to produce a narrower transmission band. A narrower bandwidth requires longer pulses, so axial resolution is degraded (although this is compensated for in part by the 2nd harmonic).

Pulse inversion: In pulse inversion (Fig. 7.32B), two pulses are transmitted: one 180° out of phase from the other. On reception, the fundamental components of the signal destructively interfere, and the 1st harmonic components constructively interfere (doubling the received amplitude), enabling imaging with the harmonic only.

This allows axial resolution to be maintained, but doubles the number of pulses required, so reducing the frame rate.

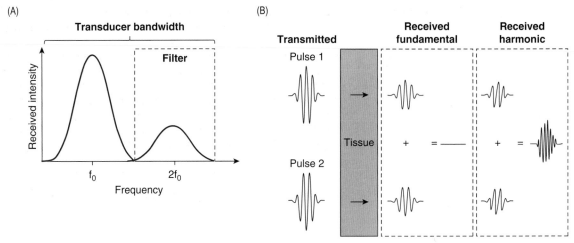

Fig. 7.32 Harmonic imaging techniques: (A) band filtering, (B) pulse inversion.

Other techniques can be used to remove the fundamental signal, including differential harmonics and amplitude modulation.

Advantages of tissue harmonic imaging include the following:

- The amplitude of the harmonic is proportional to the square of the fundamental, so small differences between signal amplitudes are enhanced. This leads to reduction or elimination of low-amplitude artefactual signals or 'clutter' such as those produced by reverberation or sidelobes.
- Different tissues produce different levels of harmonics, enhancing contrast resolution, particularly between tissue and fluid-filled cavities or cysts.

CONTRAST AGENTS

As in computed tomography and magnetic resonance imaging, contrast agents can be used in ultrasound to improve image quality and add information.

The main contrast agents used in ultrasound contain tiny, encapsulated bubbles of gas, or *microbubbles*: either air or low-solubility gas bubbles encapsulated in albumin or liquid shells. These have very low toxicity and are usually destroyed within a few hours and readily eliminated by the body, so are considered generally safe.

The diameter of microbubbles (<4 µm) is much lower than the ultrasound wavelength used but resonates at ultrasound frequencies and their harmonics. This means that microbubbles produce strong signals when they are subjected to ultrasound pulses transmitted at an appropriate frequency. The high levels of harmonics produced allow suppression of surrounding tissues by using harmonic imaging.

Commercially available contrast agents are usually produced from a solution or mixture that is agitated to produce the microbubbles and injected intravenously to examine blood flow or perfusion.

They are destroyed by higher-intensity ultrasound, so they must be imaged at lower powers. A short burst of high-intensity ultrasound can be used to destroy all the microbubbles in the field of view to study refill dynamics.

Applications include:

- Characterisation of lesion vascularity in the liver and kidneys by examining the changes in enhancement over time.
- Increasing the visibility of blood in the heart to enhance the appearance of endocardial borders.
- Assessment of peripheral vascular disease.

Other types of ultrasound contrast agent include perfluorocarbon nanoparticles for imaging of metastases or gold-bound colloidal microtubes that may be immunologically targeted. Targeted contrast agents have the potential not only for diagnosis, but also for targeted drug delivery: microbubbles are injected and then burst using a pulse of ultrasound at the target site.

DOPPLER

The Doppler effect is present whenever a sound or light wave is moving relative to the observer. When incident sound waves I of frequency f are reflected at right angles by an interface, the wavelength is altered (with speed remaining constant), depending on speed and direction of movement of the interface:

- Movement towards the transducer compresses the wave, hence wavelength decreases and frequency increases.
- Movement away from the transducer dilates the wave, hence wavelength increases and frequency decreases.

The Doppler shift $(f - f')$ is the *change* in frequency and is proportional to the velocity of the interface, v:

$$\frac{(f - f')}{f} = 2 \times \frac{v}{c}$$

hence increasing transducer frequency or speed of interface will increase Doppler shift.

Example: for $v = 30$ cm/s, $f = 10$ MHz, $c = 1540$ m/s

$$(f - f') = 2 \times f \times \frac{v}{c} = 2 \times (10 \times 10^6) \times \frac{30 \times 10^{-1}}{1540}$$

$$= 4 \text{ kHz}$$

Two aspects of the Doppler shift can be measured:

- Magnitude of change in frequency gives velocity of movement
- Measuring whether this is an increase or decrease gives the direction of movement (towards or away from the transducer)

The above refers motion in the direction of the sound only. To account for oblique angles, the term $\cos \theta$ is added (where θ is the angle of insonation — see Fig. 7.33).

$$\frac{(f - f')}{f} = 2 \times \frac{v}{c} \cos \theta$$

The maximum Doppler shift is achieved when $\cos \theta = 1$, i.e., $\theta = 0°$. For movement perpendicular to the transmitted beam, i.e., $\theta = 0°$, $\cos \theta = 0$, producing no Doppler effect.

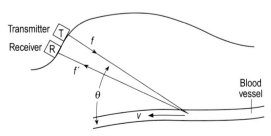

Fig. 7.33 Continuous wave Doppler: detection of blood flow in a vessel.

In diagnostic ultrasound, Doppler is usually used to measure blood flow, by measuring the signal back-scattered by blood cells.

The Doppler signal can be displayed on a screen as a spectrum, or output as audio. The Doppler shift frequency is much smaller than the transmitted frequency (within 0–10 kHz) and within the audible range, meaning that the Doppler signal can be amplified and output through a speaker: a higher pitch indicates faster flow, and a harsher sound indicates greater turbulence.

Continuous Wave (CW) Doppler

CW is the simplest form of Doppler (Fig. 7.33). Typically, it uses two slightly angled transducers: one for transmission (T), the other for reception (R). The transmitted frequency is suppressed and the Doppler shift is extracted electronically. This technique is not pulsed, so depth discrimination is not possible. Applications include monitoring the foetal heartbeat.

CW Doppler uses a high Q with no backing block to produce a precise, narrow frequency bandwidth with high output resulting in good accuracy in Doppler shift measurement. Typical frequencies used are within range of 2–10 MHz, depending on the vessel depth.

Pulsed Wave (PW) Doppler

In contrast to CW Doppler, PW Doppler enables measurement of the Doppler shift within a specified volume by using ultrasound pulses that allow depth discrimination, as for B-mode.

This technique is performed using a standard B-mode transducer, with a narrow section used for Doppler, as follows:

1. The B-mode image is produced and used to choose a line of sight for the Doppler beam.
2. Cursors along this line are chosen to define a *sampling volume*, usually positioned over the vessel in which the blood flow is to be measured (Fig. 7.34).
3. The angle of flow is specified by the user to enable accurate velocity calculation.
4. Doppler pulses are transmitted along this line to produce a Doppler signal.
5. Only echoes arriving within a short interval. The timing of this acceptance window defines the depth and width of the sampling volume, or *gate*.

Example: Ultrasound takes ~7 μs to travel 1 cm in tissue. If the range gate is opened at 70 μs and closed at 77 μs, then, accounting for the round trip:

$$70 \mu s \gg \frac{1}{2} \times \frac{70}{7} \times 1 = 5 \text{ cm}; \quad 77 \mu s \gg \frac{1}{2} \times \frac{77}{7} \times 1$$

$$= 5.5 \text{ cm}$$

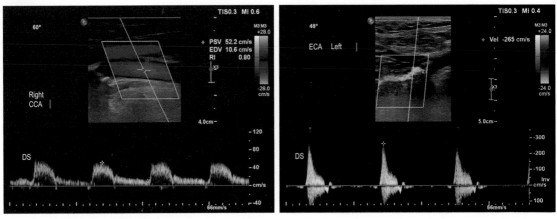

Fig. 7.34 Triplex images with the colour Doppler box superimposed onto the B-mode image, the pulsed wave Doppler range gate selected using the B-mode image, and the Doppler sonogram (DS) displayed below. Common carotid artery (CCA) on the left showing patent flow in both directions, and external carotid artery (ECA) on the right showing turbulent flow and aliasing.

Hence, blood velocities will be sampled in a volume of tissue about 5 mm thick, starting at a depth of 5 cm.

The Doppler signal comprises a wide range of audio frequencies corresponding to the range of blood velocities in the sampling volume. This can be analysed and displayed as a time-velocity spectrum or sonogram (Fig. 7.35). The transmitted Doppler frequency is used to maximise resolution, as lower frequencies allow faster flow to be measured.

Like in B-mode, the PRF depth and depth range are balanced:

- A higher PRF is used for more superficial vessels.
- The PRF is reduced as the range is increased to ensure that successive pulses do not overlap.

Real-Time Colour Flow

Whereas a greyscale (B-mode) image shows the strength of echo coming from each pixel, a *colour-mapped Doppler* image shows the direction and speed of movement or flow occurring in each pixel. The Doppler pulse is longer than that used in B-mode and the time along each line allows fewer pulses per line than PW Doppler (around 4–12 consecutive pulses in colour versus 100 in PW), so that a compromise is made between depth discrimination and accuracy of flow measurement. For this reason:

- The colour Doppler image usually covers a smaller field of view and has lower spatial resolution than the B-mode image.
- The data only allow estimation of the mean and variance (as a measure of turbulence) of velocity in each sample volume and to colour each pixel accordingly.

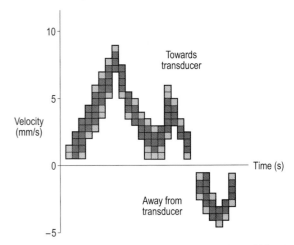

Fig. 7.35 Sonogram, showing range of velocities within the sampling volume.

The colour map is superimposed onto a user-defined region of the greyscale B-mode image using a colour scale to denote direction and speed, for example:

- Flow towards the transducer: red
- Flow away from the transducer: blue
- High-flow variance (often indicating turbulence): yellow or cyan

The performance of colour Doppler is limited by the short time available to collect the data from each beam position. The following factors can be varied and are interrelated, so should be carefully balanced:

- Frame rate, which should be fast enough to follow changes in flow velocity.
- Penetration depth, which is inversely proportional to PRF.
- Field width, or sector which can be reduced to increase frame rate.
- Line density, which should be high enough for good spatial resolution.
- PRF, which can be controlled using the colour scale and should be high enough to give accurate velocity information.

The combinations of two or three imaging methods such as B-mode and PW Doppler and/or colour Doppler are known as *duplex or triplex imaging,* respectively. This is achieved by transmitting bursts of Doppler pulses between B-mode pulses.

Doppler Aliasing

In pulsed Doppler modes, the Doppler shift is measured by detecting the phase of successive pulses. To accurately measure the full range of frequencies in this way, the sampling rate must be high enough to satisfy the Nyquist criterion, i.e., the PRF must satisfy:

$$PRF \geq f_{max}$$

Where f_{max} is the maximum Doppler shift in the sampled volume. High-velocity flow outside of this limit therefore results in aliasing, manifesting as flow in the opposite direction. This appears as follows:

- In PW Doppler, the top of the spectrum wraps around from the top to the bottom of the trace (or vice versa).
- On colour Doppler, flow that should appear red changes to black and then blue. Fast laminar flow appears as an aliased blue centre with a red edge (or vice versa) and high-speed jets with associated turbulence appear as a coloured mosaic.

Aliasing can be resolved by increasing the Doppler scale to increase the PRF, or by switching to CW Doppler, which does not suffer from aliasing.

If a high enough PRF is not possible at the depth of flow examined, this can be partially overcome using high PRF mode. As in Fig. 7.36, instead of only sampling from a single volume A, doubling the PRF samples in both volume A and another at half the depth, B. Increasing the PRF further samples from even more volumes. This method relies on appropriate positioning by the operator to ensure that only one sample volume is positioned over an area of flow.

Power Doppler

Power Doppler images do not give any indication of speed or direction, but instead maps the *amplitude* of the

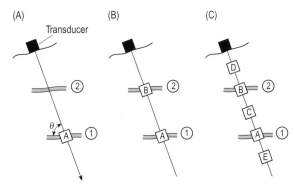

Fig. 7.36 Pulsed Doppler: (A) normal and (B and C) high pulse repetition frequency modes; 1 and 2 are blood vessels.

Doppler signal. A higher density of red blood cells produces a greater amplitude signal, which appears brighter on the image. In this case, all movement, regardless of phase, contributes to the amplitude, so the power Doppler image reflects the *quantity* of blood flow.

The main application of power Doppler is to differentiate between areas with and without flow, often where the flow is slow, like in imaging vessel walls. It is also much more sensitive than colour Doppler, enabling imaging of smaller vessels and perfusion of organs such as the kidneys. This technique does not suffer from aliasing as it does not measure velocity, but its high sensitivity does make it susceptible to artefacts caused by the motion of surrounding tissue.

ELASTOGRAPHY

As well as imaging, ultrasound can be used to examine the elasticity or stiffness of tissues. There are two main techniques: strain imaging and shear wave elastography.

Strain imaging: Ultrasound imaging is performed before and during compression of the tissue, using either:
1. Free-hand compression
2. Mechanical compression
3. Internal physiological movement such as cardiovascular or respiratory
4. Acoustic radiation force impulse (ARFI): using a short, high-intensity ultrasound pulse to produce a radiation force that causes tissue displacement

The tissue displacement caused by the applied stress is estimated to determine the deformation (i.e., stiffer tissues deform less than more elastic tissues). This is used to produce a colour map of strain distribution, showing tissue hardness, which is superimposed onto a B-mode image. Because it is not possible to quantify the stress applied in techniques 1–3, these produce qualitative results and cannot be used for absolute measurement of tissue stiffness.

Shear wave elastography: The speed of sound depends on tissue stiffness, therefore by measuring the speed, the stiffness can be quantified. Shear waves travel much more slowly in soft tissue than longitudinal compression waves: approximately 1–10 m/s. This allows the shear wave propagation to be imaged as it propagates (usually with A-mode ultrasound), allowing its speed to be calculated. Ultrasound imaging is performed before and during the generation of shear waves in the tissue, using either:
1. Mechanical vibration of the probe
2. ARFI

The calculated shear wave speed is converted to a quantitative measure of tissue stiffness. Depending on the technique employed, this can be done using A-mode or B-mode, to produce a quantitative measurement for a chosen area, or two-dimensional colour map.

SAFETY CONSIDERATIONS

Ultrasound is not an electromagnetic radiation and is non-ionising. Used in diagnosis, it is a low-risk and low-cost method of medical imaging. However, harmful biological effects have been identified at exposure levels more usually associated with ultrasound therapy.

There has been no confirmed evidence of damage from diagnostic ultrasound exposure. However, the output of each probe should be checked periodically, and operators should keep within safety guidelines (see below), to minimise the potential for effects such as the following:

Thermal effects:

Local heating due to frictional, viscous, and molecular relaxation processes, leading to chemical damage but mitigated by blood flow. The risk from this effect is increased for patients who already have a raised body temperature, or in more sensitive tissues including the embryo; the head, brain, or spine of a foetus or neonate; and the eye.

Mechanical/Nonthermal Effects

- **Cavitation:** The high peak pressure changes can cause microbubbles in a liquid or near liquid medium to oscillate (expand and contract). If the expansion results in very sudden collapse (inertial cavitation), this can cause cellular damage. This is more likely at high pressures and low frequencies and if pulses are long enough to allow resonance to be reached. It is also more likely in the presence of existing gas such as in the lung or bowel or when using microbubble contrast agents.

- Acoustic streaming of cellular contents in the direction of the beam, affecting cell membrane permeability.
- Mechanical damage to cell membranes caused by violent acceleration of particles.

Output Measures and Safety Indices

The intensity of an ultrasound beam is greatest in the focal region. Typically, the time-averaged intensity (I_{SPTA}: the spatial peak averaged over the examination) is around 0.1 W/mm^2. The peak intensity (I_{SPTP}: the intensity at the time during the brief pulse when it is at the peak) is likely to be 1000 times greater. The I_{SPTA} will increase for longer pulses, such as those used in Doppler.

Thermal effects are estimated using the thermal index (TI), which gives an indication of the temperature rise in tissue:

$$TI = \frac{\textit{Emitted Power}}{\textit{Power required to increase the temperature by 1°C}}$$

As the TI increases above the value of 1, exposure times should be reduced appropriately, depending on the application and the condition of the patient. Recommended exposure times are given by the British Medical Ultrasound Society,[1] along with a summary of ultrasound safety and techniques for exposure reduction. For example, scanning at a TI of 2.0 can be performed for up to 60 min, whereas at a TI of 3.0, times should be restricted to 4 min. Further care and more restrictive scan times are needed in obstetric or ophthalmic imaging or when the patient is feverish.

Mechanical effects are estimated using the mechanical index (MI): the maximum amplitude of the pressure pulse, defined as the peak rarefaction (negative) pressure divided by the square root of the ultrasound frequency. As with TI, exam times should be reduced appropriately once MI reaches the threshold of 0.7, at which mechanical effects are thought to occur.

Diagnostic ultrasound equipment output should not exceed the following:
- Derated $I_{SPTA} \leq 720$ mW/cm^2 (this is further reduced for applications such as cardiac, foetal, or ophthalmic imaging)
- MI ≤ 1.9 or derated $I_{SPTA} \leq 190$ W/kg

The calculated indices, MI and TI, which are worst-case-based, should be indicated on the scanner display when the equipment is capable of exceeding an index value of 1, to enable users to continuously monitor exposure and reduce scan times accordingly.

QUALITY ASSURANCE

Ultrasound scanners are generally reliable and stable; however, slight damage to a probe or drift in the electronics can lead to deterioration of the image. Image quality tests to detect faults include the following:

- **Sensitivity:** tested by imaging in air to produce a reverberation image. A reduction in the depth of the last reverberation is an indication of a reduction in sensitivity.
- **Low contrast penetration and uniformity:** tested by imaging a uniform tissue-mimicking material (TMM). Penetration is determined by measuring the depth at which the speckle produced from the TMM is no longer visible. Examining the uniformity of the image can detect other faults such as a broken transducer element.
- **Spatial resolution:** tested by imaging narrow threads or pin targets mounted on a frame and immersed in a fluid in which the speed of sound is 1540 m/s, and measuring the spread axially and laterally of the cross-section. Imaging the spread of these pins allows a rough visualisation of the variation in in-plane beam width with depth and rotating the probe surface by 45°.
- Other image quality tests such as greyscale performance and Doppler function require more complex test objects, often in a TMM containing test objects of varying dimensions and acoustic properties (Fig. 7.37).

The power output of the transducer is measured by 'weighing' the sound pressure with a force balance or by measuring the heating effect using a calorimeter. More sophisticated techniques can be used to measure the

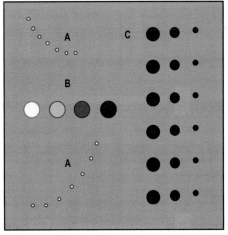

Fig. 7.37 Example tissue-mimicking test object containing targets for measuring (A) resolution, (B) greyscale performance, and (C) anechoic target detection.

intensity or pressure distribution throughout the ultrasound field.

Recommendations for routine quality assurance are given by the Institute of Physics and Engineering in Medicine in Report 102.[2]

REFERENCES

1. British Medical Ultrasound Society. *Guidelines for the Safe Use of Diagnostic Ultrasound Equipment.* London, UK: BMUS; 2009.
2. Institute of Physics and Engineering in Medicine. *Report 102: Quality Assurance of Ultrasound Imaging Systems.* York, UK: IPEM; 2010.

8

Radiology Information Technology

CHAPTER CONTENTS

The digital world is defined by the quantisation of data. All information (e.g., the values for a given image) is represented by discrete finite values. Quantisation of information is ubiquitous in our modern world and has allowed the interaction of medical data with specialities and fields of research that would not have previously been considered. One of the biggest challenges to radiology is storage of the ever-increasing sizes of data acquired with each imaging event. The way this data is stored, communicated, and processed will be outlined in this chapter.

IMAGE MATRIX

- The information in a radiological exposure is recorded to a matrix
  - For 2D radiology (e.g., X-ray/2D ultrasound) this yields a 2D matrix of rows and columns consisting of pixels (picture elements, see Fig. 8.1)
  - For 3D radiology (e.g., computed tomography [CT] and magnetic resonance imaging [MRI]), this yields a 3D matrix of voxels (volume elements)
    - The 3D volume acquired (usually a cuboid shape) has been quantised into smaller voxels (Fig. 8.2)
    - If the voxels are cubes, they are considered isotropic
    - If the Z-axis of the voxel is different, these are anisotropic
      - X-Y axis size for pixels or voxels is always the same as the detector elements used to acquire the information in a square

- See Fig. 8.3
- The amount of information per element is determined by the bit depth
  - Bit depth $= 2^n$, where n is the number of bits allocated to memory available in binary format
  - This indicates the range of values for a given element
    - Bit depth of 12 yields 4096 possible value levels
    - See Fig. 8.4
    - Increased bit depth increases data size
- For a bit depth of 2, there are 4 levels recordable
  - Values 0–3 available
  - A value of 0 is recorded not as 0, but 00
  - A value of 3 is recorded not as 3, but 11
- Image fusion
  - Some modalities (e.g., positron emission tomography [PET]-CT, PET MRI) fuse the information from two different acquisitions to create a single image
    - See Fig. 8.5
  - The greyscale CT/MRI is used as the base image
  - Overlayed onto this is the PET imaging information using a colour map display format
    - Uses a transparency value (α)
    - The value of α is governed by the voxel values of the PET
  - Low voxel values (areas of limited PET uptake) use an α level near 0, and have little impact on the base CT/MRI image

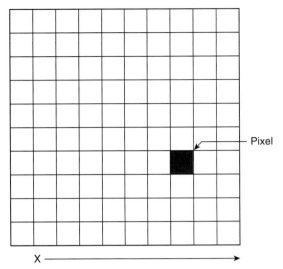

Fig. 8.1 Graphical representation of a 2D matrix of pixels.

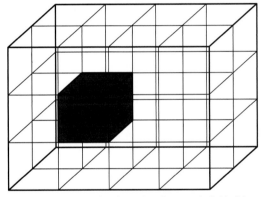

Fig. 8.2 Cuboid-imaged volume has been subdivided into 24 isotropic voxels.

- High voxel values (areas of high PET uptake) use an α level near 1, and saturate the image with colour
  - The voxel sizes of PET images are usually much larger than CT/MRI, hence the areas of colour seem block-like and pixelated
  - The position of each voxel of the CT/MRI image relative to the PET image is governed by patient position data stored in the Digital Imaging and Communications in Medicine (DICOM) file
- If the patient moves, there is misregistration of the two datasets and the voxels do not overlap accurately
- See Fig. 8.6
Also see Box 8.1.

DISPLAY

- LCD screens are now standard
  - High spatial resolution
  - Low distortion
  - High luminance
  - High contrast ratio
  - Reduced energy consumption
- CRT is obsolete
- Differing requirements for the setup for the radiologist for primary reporting compared with clinical reviews
- DICOM greyscale standard display function (GSDF)
  - Means to generate a lookup table (LUT) to produce consistent perceptible shades of grey
  - Maps and monitors digital driving levels
  - Requires quality control
  - For primary diagnostics – 10% DICOM GSDF required over lifetime of display
  - For clinical review – 20% DICOM GSDF required over lifetime of display
  - Mobile devices cannot be calibrated but can be tested for suitability
- Standard red, green, and blue (sRGB) is recommended for colour requirements
  - The colour maps applied convert the greyscale data to colour based on a variety of RGB lookup tables
  - Used to make subtle differences more apparent to the human observer
  - There are 256 individual values available for red, green, and blue which produce the spectrum of colour when combined
  - At present, a colour standard display function has been proposed, but is not yet adopted
- Dedicated medical display (DMD) vs consumer-grade off-the-shelf (COTS)
  - DMDs include self-calibration and quality control to ensure drift and deterioration of DICOM GSDF do not occur over lifetime
  - COTS suitable for clinical review devices
- The most stringent requirements are in mammography:
  - 5-megapixel minimum resolution (2560 × 2048 pixels)
  - Pixel pitch maximum is 170 μm
  - DICOM GSDF ≤10% at all times
  - Luminance 1/400 cd/m^2
    - cd = Candela (SI unit of luminous intensity)

IMAGE DATA

DICOM represents the international standard for medical imaging and related information (ISO 12052). Conversion of acquired raw image data to DICOM format occurs at each computer modality. It is important to note that, for

(A)

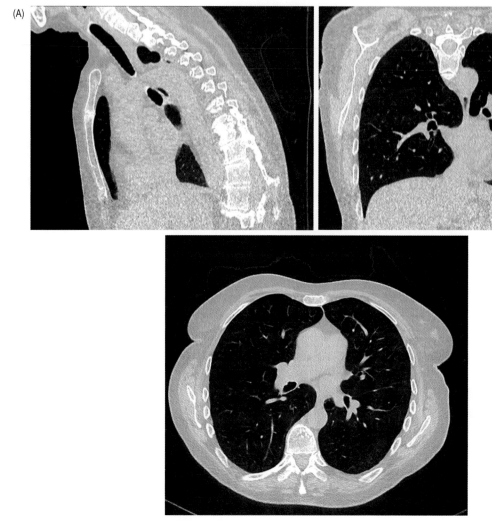

Fig. 8.3 (A) Isotropic voxels with the same in-plane resolution in transaxial, coronal, and sagittal views.

certain modalities with large raw datasets (e.g., CT), only specified reconstructions of the data in DICOM format are transferred to the picture archiving and communication system (PACS).

Consists of:

- Header file
  - Contains the metadata for each corresponding DICOM image
    - Diverse range of entries possible
      - Not all entries are used for every examination
      - Not all entries necessary for function of the DICOM image
      - Format (xxxx, yyyy)
      - E.g. (0010, 0010) — Patient's name

- If xxxx is an odd number, this is likely a manufacturer-added private-key entry and not necessarily part of the DICOM dictionary standard
- Enables the accurate and consistent display of images between devices and workstations
  - Ensures the correct image set is associated with the correct patient for a specified time point
    - Allows separation of patient imaging by time-point and modality
  - Enables DICOM display software to accurately display images
    - Each slice in an MRI sequence is displayed sequentially, with only slices from that

(B)

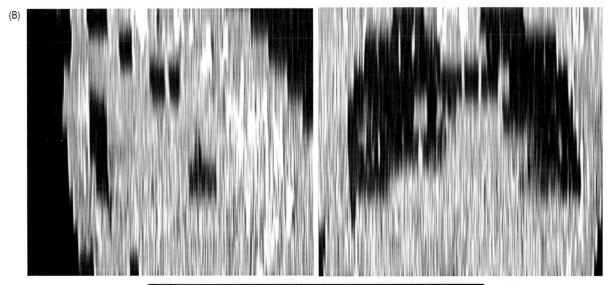

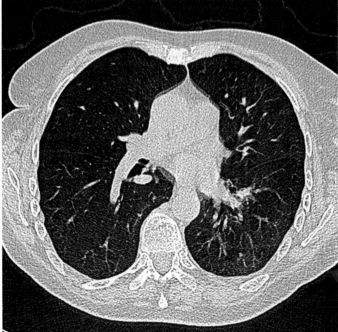

Fig. 8.3 cont'd. (B) Anisotropic voxels with different transaxial and Z-axis voxel dimensions (coronal and sagittal views have limited use).

sequence, and can be cross-referenced with alternative planes of imaging

- Acquired CT volume can be interrogated as a 3D object with varying angles of orientation or slice thickness

- Separately acquired PET and CT images can be fused together to form a hybrid image
- Ensures that the default image display parameters are the same (governed by any postprocessing performed)

Pixel value

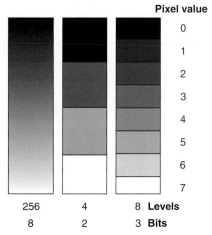

| 256 | 4 | 8 **Levels** |
| 8 | 2 | 3 **Bits** |

Fig. 8.4 Greyscales with different bit depths.

- Some example header information: (all can be accessed for each DICOM image using either a meta-data reader, or DICOM information/elements functionality on the PACS)
  - Hardware/software parameters
    - Type of scan (CT, X-ray [XR], computed radiography [CR], digital radiography [DR], nuclear medicine NM), MR, X-ray angiography [XA], ultrasound [US], PET [PT], other [OT], mammography [MG])
    - Scanner used, institution, time of acquisition
- All have unique identifiers
  - Patient-specific identifiers
    - Name, date of birth, sex, age (at time of acquisition), smoking history, pregnancy status, contrast allergy, address, occupation, religious affiliation

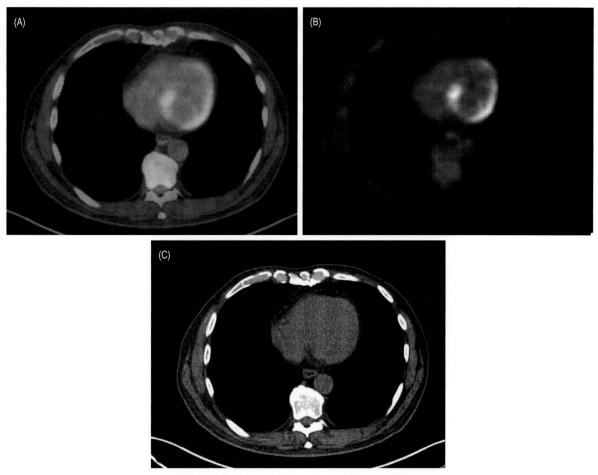

Fig. 8.5 (A) Transaxial image of a fused positron emission tomography (PET)/computed tomography (CT) image at the level of the heart. (B) The standard PET image. (C) The base CT image.

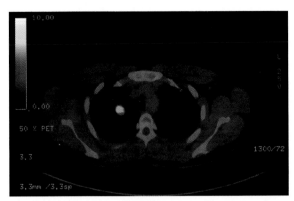

Fig. 8.6 Misregistration of images. The computed tomography and positron emission tomography (PET) images of the right upper lobe lung nodule do not fully overlap, likely secondary to breathing in this instance. This image shows the standard 'hot iron' colour map used to display the PET images.

- Acquisition parameters
  - MR sequence (e.g., field strength, repetition time, phase-encoding steps, echo time, flip angle)
  - Radiopharmaceutical information

- Slice location, position information (to allow formation of a 3D image)
- Pixel size, pixel values (low/high), rows/columns per image, resolution
- Magnification
- Dose
  - Tube current, exposure time
  - Dose-area product/dose-length product
  - Phantom used for quality assurance (QA)
  - Combined to form a radiation dose structured report (see below)
- Postprocessing
  - LUT applied, window centre/width applied
  - Compression
- Anonymisation
  - Extensive manipulation and deletion of elements of the metadata is required to enable full anonymisation of a DICOM image
  - Some DICOM images have patient data present in the image data which may need manual manipulation to remove
- Image data
  - Individual stored values of each pixel/voxel
  - Range of values depends on the modality

BOX 8.1   1D Fourier Analysis

In an ideal system, there is instantaneous delineation of the boundary at a discrete edge (Fig. 8.7A). Every system has limitations, after which there is blurring of the edges, often defined as spatial frequency (expressed as line pairs per mm or cycles per mm). The system limitations are determined by evaluating the impulse response function of the detectors (Fig. 8.7B). Fourier analysis allows a function to be interrogated and re-represented as a series of known simpler trigonometric functions in the modulation transfer function (Fig. 8.7C).

The square wave (A) in Fig. 8.8 represents the pattern of X-rays produced in an ideal imaging system scanning across Fig. 8.9. The peak value represents the gap between the lead bars, and the trough the lead bars. A sine wave (B) with the same spatial frequency is drawn onto the graph. The amplitude, or peak-to-peak height, has been adjusted so that the area below the sine wave is equal to that below the square wave. The sine wave is a poor representation of the original. A closer fit may be achieved by adding a second sine wave with 3 times the spatial frequency and one-third the amplitude (profile C). Successive additions of sine waves with 5, 7, and 9 times

the frequency and one-fifth, one-seventh, and one-ninth of the amplitude and so on will provide an increasingly closer fit to the square wave. Profile D in the figure goes up to the sine wave with 15 times the spatial frequency and one-fifteenth of the amplitude. Note that only odd numbers are used in this mathematical technique. Continuing up to an infinite series would produce a perfect reproduction of the original.

The signal produced by scanning across a single narrow strip of lead can similarly be analysed into a spectrum of sine waves, but now the spectrum contains a wider range of frequencies, and the higher frequencies have more amplitude. The narrower the strip, the wider the band of sine wave frequencies involved and the more important the high frequencies. This is what is meant by saying that a fine structure with a sharp edge is composed of or corresponds to high spatial frequencies, whereas a large diffuse structure is composed of or corresponds only to low frequencies. To reproduce small, sharp structures in the image, the system has to be able to handle high spatial frequencies without loss of signal or contrast.

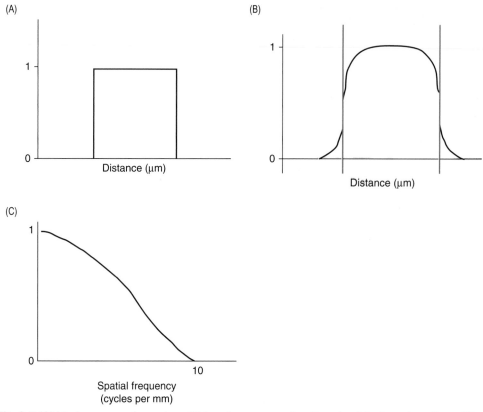

Fig. 8.7 (A) Ideal response of a system. (B) Impulse response function of a detector, where the red lines indicate the boundaries of the input impulse. (C) Modulation transfer function.

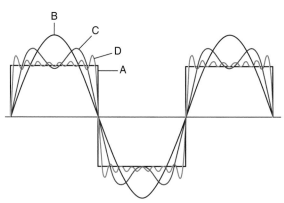

Fig. 8.8 1D Fourier analysis of A, a square waveform that can be represented by B, a single sine wave, C, the sum of two sine waves, or D, a function with eight sine wave components.

Fig. 8.9 Resolution grid.

- For 16-bit storage, over 65,000 possible levels are available; however, modalities are often displayed in the following ranges:
  - CT [−2000 +3000] HU
  - X-ray [0 4095]
  - MRI [0 5000]
- For fluoroscopy, there is only 8-bit depth, so the levels are at 0−256
- The relationship between each pixel/voxel is determined by the information contained in the metadata

Radiation Dose Structured Report

- Mechanism for tracking and recording the radiation dose for each examination
- This report is exported as a DICOM image attached to the main imaging encounter (Figs. 8.10 and 8.11). For X-ray (CR/DR), the report information is contained in the metadata alone

- Prior to the implementation of this report, dose data was directly attached to each image. If an image was not stored, the record of the dose was lost
- Dose information (e.g., CT dose index-volume) is based on the equivalent dose for the phantom used in QA for that machine, not a patient-specific dose

Compression

- DICOM images are data-heavy file types, especially when considered at the magnitude and scale of diagnostic imaging
  - A single MG/CR/DR image can be >30 MB
  - A single US image is between 0.8−1 MB, but there may be 25 images per scan
  - A single 2D MR image is usually <200 kB, but there may be 1400 images per scan
  - A single CT image is 0.5−0.7 MB, but there can be >2000 images for a triple-phase scan

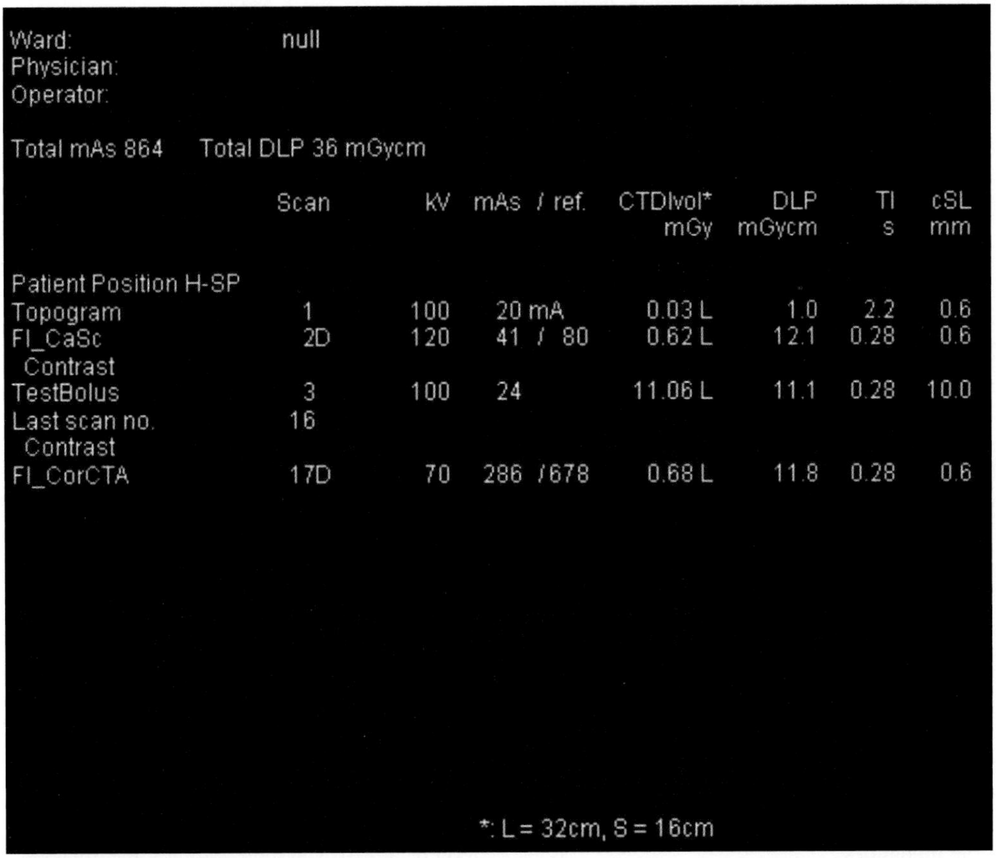

	Scan	kV	mAs / ref.	CTDIvol* mGy	DLP mGycm	TI s	cSL mm
Ward:	null						
Physician:							
Operator:							
Total mAs 864	Total DLP 36 mGycm						
Patient Position H-SP							
Topogram	1	100	20 mA	0.03 L	1.0	2.2	0.6
Fl_CaSc	2D	120	41 / 80	0.62 L	12.1	0.28	0.6
Contrast							
TestBolus	3	100	24	11.06 L	11.1	0.28	10.0
Last scan no.	16						
Contrast							
Fl_CorCTA	17D	70	286 /678	0.68 L	11.8	0.28	0.6

*: L = 32cm, S = 16cm

Fig. 8.10 Radiation dose structured report for a computed tomography examination. The total mAs and dose-length product (DLP) are shown at the top. A breakdown of the kV, mAs parameters, and doses for each component are also shown.

```
                              Exam Protocol
-----------------------------------------------------------------------------------
Patient Info:
Name:
-----------------------------------------------------------------------------------
Patient Position:  HFS

1    DSA            FIXED     Extr.2 CARE              12s    2F/s
A  63kV  377mA  139.5ms  0.0CL small 0.6Cu 48cm  277.41µGym²  6.4mGy   0LAO   0CRA   23F

2    DSA            FIXED     Extr.2 CARE              12s    2F/s
A  65kV  406mA  144.2ms  0.0CL small 0.6Cu 48cm  224.29µGym²  9.7mGy   17RAO  0CRA   23F

3    DSA            FIXED     Extr.2 CARE              10s    2F/s
A  66kV  408mA  144.3ms  0.0CL small 0.6Cu 48cm  194.85µGym²  8.1mGy   17RAO  0CRA   19F

4    DSA            FIXED     Extr.2 CARE               7s    2F/s
A  65kV  405mA  143.1ms  0.0CL small 0.6Cu 48cm  102.09µGym²  5.5mGy   16LAO  0CRA   13F

5    DSA            FIXED     Extr.2 CARE               7s    2F/s
A  66kV  408mA   91.5ms  0.0CL small 0.3Cu 48cm  174.21µGym²  9.4mGy   16LAO  10CRA  13F

6    DSA            FIXED     Extr.2 CARE               7s    2F/s
A  66kV  408mA  106.2ms  0.0CL small 0.3Cu 48cm  217.92µGym²  11.7mGy  16LAO  10CRA  14F

7    DSA            FIXED     Extr.2 CARE               8s    2F/s
A  67kV  419mA  141.0ms  0.1CL small 0.3Cu 48cm  337.59µGym²  18.2mGy  29LAO  10CRA  15F

8    DSA            FIXED     Extr.2 CARE               8s    2F/s
A  67kV  415mA  141.0ms  0.1CL small 0.3Cu 48cm  349.35µGym²  18.8mGy  29LAO  10CRA  16F

***Accumulated exposure data***
Performing Physician:                         Exposures: 8
Total Fluoro: 00:16:44                        Total: 2296.3µGym²    109.4mGy
A     Fluoro: 00:16:44    418.59µGym²   21.7mGy   Total: 2296.3µGym²    109.4mGy

===================================================================================
-----------------------------------------------------------------------------------
```

Fig. 8.11 Radiation dose structured report for a fluoroscopy examination. The kV, mA, dose, time, and table position of each run is shown. At the bottom is a summation of total time and dose.

- In view of this demand on hardware (data storage, transfer, and image display), some form of compression is desired
- Lossy compression
  - Higher compression ratio (8:1–30:1)
  - Irreversible compression algorithm
  - Limited to a level not to affect diagnostic performance
- Lossless
  - Fully reversible compression
  - Ratios of 2:1 or 3:1 possible

PACS

PACS — technological system for:
- Storage and convenient access to images
  - Secure network
  - Multiple modalities
  - Replaces physical copy archives
- Backup facilities
- Same images can be viewed simultaneously in different locations
- Archive storage/retrieval
- Reading apparatus (dedicated workstations for primary reporting or web browser based for clinical review)
- Integration with other systems
  - Hospital information systems
  - Radiology information systems
  - Electronic medical record
  - Communication protocol standards
    - HL-7 (health level 7)
    - DICOM
- The overall system is overviewed in Fig. 8.12.

RADIOLOGY INFORMATION SYSTEM

Where a PACS system handles the imaging data for a radiology system, the radiology information system (RIS)

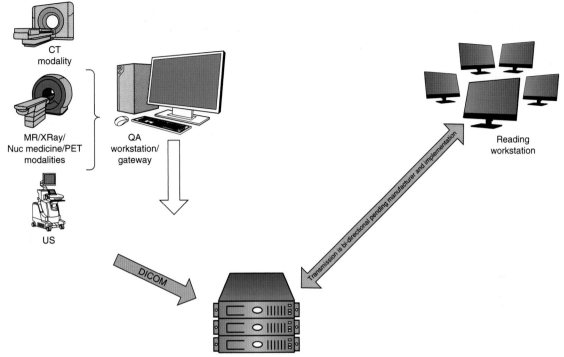

Fig. 8.12 Picture Archiving and Communication System (PACS) overview.

manages the remainder of the functions in a radiology system. This includes, but is not limited to:

- Patient requests
  - Provides an interface for clinicians to request a radiological study
    - With the facility for scanned paper requests (used during system downtime)
  - Assigns each request for a given patient to a specific electronic entry
  - Provides a mechanism for the radiologist/practitioner to justify and authorise a radiological study or to return the request to the clinician
  - Enables the operator to perform the study after authorisation
  - Couples the DICOM stored in PACS with the specific electronic entry
- Patient reporting
  - Provides a workflow for the reporter to assess the current images for a patient along with request history, and any previous examinations available for that patient
  - Voice recognition software

- Mechanisms for communication of urgent reports to responsible clinician
  - PACS-based reporting is also available
- Workflow management
  - Co-ordination of modality worklists
  - Co-ordination of patient appointments
    - A+E/Inpatient
    - Outpatient urgent/routine
- Integration with hospital information systems

FURTHER READING

European Society of Radiology. Usability of irreversible image compression in radiological imaging. A position paper by the European Society of Radiology (ESR). *Insights Imaging.* 2011; 2:103−115.

Royal College of Radiologists. *Picture Archiving and Communication Systems (PACS) and Guidelines on Diagnostic Display Devices.* 3rd ed. London, UK: The Royal College of Radiologists; 2019.

Santos DPD, others. The impact of irreversible image data compression on post-processing algorithms in computed tomography. *Diagn Interv Radiol.* 2020;26:22−27.

Allisy-Roberts P, Williams J. *Farr's Physics for Medical Imaging.* 2nd ed. UK: WB Saunders Company; 2008.

British Institute of Radiology. *Assurance of Quality in the Diagnostic Imaging Department.* 2nd ed. London: BIR; 2003.

Cherry SR, Sorenson J, Phelps M. *Physics in Nuclear Medicine.* 3rd ed. Philadelphia: Saunders; 2003.

Curry TS, Dowdey JE, Murry RC. *Christensen's Physics of Diagnostic Radiology.* 4th ed. Philadelphia: Lea & Febiger; 1990.

Dendy PP, Heaton B. *Physics for Diagnostic Radiology.* 2nd ed. Bristol: Institute of Physics Publishing; 1999.

Health and Safety Commission. *Work With Ionising Radiation L121 (Ionising Radiations Regulations 1999, Approved Code of Practice and Guidance).* London: Health and Safety Executive; 2000.

Hendee WR, Ritenour ER. *Medical Imaging Physics.* 4th ed. New York: Wiley-Liss; 2002.

Hendrick WR, Hykes DL, Starchman DE. *Ultrasound Physics and Instrumentation.* 4th ed. Philadelphia: Elsevier; 2005.

Institute of Physics and Engineering in Medicine. *Medical and Dental Guidance Notes: A Good Practice Guide on All Aspects of Ionising Radiation Protection in the Clinical Environment.* York: IPEM; 2002.

Institute of Physics and Engineering in Medicine. *Recommended Standards for the Routine Performance Testing of Diagnostic X-ray Imaging Systems, Report 91.* York: IPEM; 2005.

Kalender WA. *Computed Tomography: Fundamentals, System Technology, Image Quality, Applications.* 2nd ed. Erlangen: Publicis; 2005.

Martin CJ, Dendy PP, Corbett RH. *Medical Imaging and Radiation Protection for Medical Students and Clinical Staff.* London: British Institute of Radiology; 2003.

Martin CJ, Sutton DG, eds. *Practical Radiation Protection in Healthcare.* Oxford: Oxford University Press; 2002.

McRobbie DW, Moore EA, Graves MJ, Prince MR. *MRI From Picture to Proton.* Cambridge: Cambridge University Press; 2006.

Saha GB. *Basics of PET Imaging.* New York: Springer; 2004.

Tolan D, Hyland R, Taylor C, Cowen A. *FRCR Part 1: MCQs and Mock Examination.* London: Royal Society of Medicine Press; 2004.

Westbrook C. *MRI at a Glance.* Oxford: Blackwell Science; 2002.

Page numbers followed by *f* indicate figures; *t*, tables; and *b*, boxes.

A

absorbed dose, 6b
absorption edges, photoelectric effect, 10
acoustic impedance (Z), 149, 149t
acoustic matching, ultrasound, 154
acoustic radiation force impulse (ARFI), 171
acoustic shadowing/enhancement, ultrasound, 166, 167f
acquisition camera, 99
acquisition parameters, 112—113
  matrix of, 112
  motion of, 113
  patient factors in, 113
  projection views of, 112—113
acquisition time, image, 110
active-pixel sensor, for CCD, 63
ADC map. *See* apparent diffusion coefficient map
air gap, 43, 43f
aliasing, pulsed Doppler ultrasound, 171
aliasing artefact, 132, 132f
alpha particles, 3t, 15
aluminium, 3t, 20
amplification, of photomultiplier tubes, 98
angular range, 112—113
angular step, 112
anode, 98, 98f
  X-ray tube, 4
anode heel effect, 43f
APDs. *See* avalanche photodiodes
apparent diffusion coefficient (ADC) map, 144, 144t
Approved Code of Practice (ACOP), radiation protection, 31
approved dosimetry service, Ionising Radiations Regulations (1999), 33
ARFI. *See* acoustic radiation force impulse
arm position, in acquisition parameters, 113
array, types of, 72, 73f
artefacts
  chemical shift
    phase cancellation, 135—136, 137f
    spatial misregistration, 135, 136f

artefacts (*Continued*)
  cross-talk, 130—132, 132f
  dielectric, 141
  Dixon, 136, 137f
  flow, 141, 141f
  k-space, 139
  metal, 141, 142f
  of MRI, 140—141
  parallel imaging, 140
  wrap/aliasing, 132, 132f
  zipper, 141, 142f
arterial spin labelling (ASL), 145
as low as reasonably achievable (ALARA), radiation protection, 30
as low as reasonably practicable (ALARP), radiation protection, 30
ASL. *See* arterial spin labelling
atomic number, 1, 8
atomic structure, 1—2, 2f
attenuation, of gamma radiation, 115
  analytical, 115
  direct measurement of, 115
attenuation coefficient, linear, 8
automatic brightness control, for fluoroscopy, 64, 65f
auto-ranging, in image processing, 49
avalanche photodiodes (APDs), 120
axial (depth) resolution, ultrasound, 163, 163f

B

B_1 inhomogeneities, 141
B_{1+} RMS, 127
back projection, 113, 113f
band filtering, ultrasound, 167, 168f
bandwidth, 150
barium fluoride, physical properties of, 117t
beta emission, 15
binding energy, 2, 3t
bismuth germinate, physical properties of, 117, 117t
blood cell labelling, 18
bow-tie filter, 70, 72f
Bragg curve, 12f
breast tomosynthesis, 56—58, 60f—61f

C

cadmium-zinc-telluride (CZT), 99—100
calcium, 3t

cardiac black-blood imaging, 138
cardiac CT/gated imaging, 88—90, 88f—89f, 91f
cartesian filling, of k-space, 139f
cast collimators, 97
cathode, X-ray tube, 4
cavitation, ultrasound, 172
characteristic radiation
  photoelectric effect, 10
  X-ray production, 7f, 10
charge coupled device (CCD), 48
  for fluoroscopy, 63, 64f
charged particles, 11—12
chemical compound, addition to, 18
chemical purity, 20
chemical-shift misregistration artefact, 135, 136f
classified persons, Ionising Radiations Regulations (1999), 33
CNR. *See* contrast-to-noise ratio
coincidence detection, of PET, 118
collimator, 96—98
  in acquisition parameters, 113
  indicative values of, 105t
  Medical and Dental Guidance Notes, 31
  resolution, 102—103
  in SPECT, 112
  types of, 97f
comforters and carers, 35
  dose limits, 30
compressed sensing (CS), 139
Compton scatter (effect), 9—10, 10f
  electron density, 10, 10f
  photoelectric effect *vs.*, 10, 11f
computed radiography (CR), 44—45, 46f—47f
computed tomography (CT), 69—95
  additional capabilities of, 88—93, 88f—89f, 91f
  applications of, 91f—92f
  artefacts, 80—82, 81f—82f, 82b
  basics of, 69, 70f, 71b
  components used in image acquisition of, 70—72, 72f
  contrast, 80
  detectors of, 71
  dose, 93—95, 93f—94f
  image acquisition of, 72—74